"I was FAT at age 3. I'm now a 55-year-old woman, morbidly obese, and my body is telling me 'Beware!'. I've mastered self-denial, and have created workable, reasonable justifications for my lifestyle. After all, 'I am The FAT KID'". Since reading Julie's book, I've freed myself from this story. I've learned that change does not start with what I'm eating, how I'm exercising, or what size I am. Change starts with how I think about food and my body. For the first time ever, I'm actually IN my body. I listen to its needs and desires and no longer feel I'm depriving it. I eat the foods I want with emotional and personal balance, and I'm still losing weight! This is a life-alerting change, and Julie's book has been a huge part of this. Kudos, my dear friend!

Garnett Stewart, *R.N., M.S.*

Today's society has created and fostered the proliferation of obesity. And while the get-thin-quick industry is failing, Julie Hammerstein hits the nail on the head with ***Fat Is Not A Four-Letter Word.*** Julie harnesses the most powerful force available in the pursuit of a wellness-centered life; the muscle between your ears. Simple and straightforward writing from personal experience makes this a valuable weight-loss resource at a time when we need it most.

Wade Perry, *Dad, Husband, Entrepreneur, Wellness Seeker*

FAT

IS NOT A FOUR-LETTER WORD

**14 Daily Lessons to Break Through
Your "Fat Kid Mentality"
and Keep The Weight Off for Life!**

Julie Hammerstein, CN

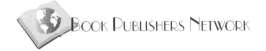

BOOK PUBLISHERS NETWORK

Book Publishers Network
P. O. Box 2256
Bothell, WA 98041
425 483-3040
www.bookpublishersnetwork.com

10 9 8 7 6 5 4 3 2 1

LCCN 2010915013
ISBN 10 1-935359-56-8
ISBN 13 978-1-935359-56-2

Editor: Vicki McCown
Cover designer: Laura Zugzda
Typographer: Nina Barnett

This book is dedicated to my grandparents, Susan and Frank Kelly, Chester and Grace Hammerstein, and Jim and Pat Rheem.

I feel your presence, and I am grateful for your guidance. You taught me how to live in the world with grace, confidence and unconditional love.

And to my aunt, Barbara Bates ("Suti"), who introduced me to poetry and who shared a deep love of the written word.

FOREWORD

We were thrilled to write the foreword to this book for several reasons. Not only is it flattering to be called on to endorse Julie's work; it is above all, exciting and encouraging to see more authors empowering people to ditch the diets and embrace a new approach to weight-loss and body confidence.

When our book, *Beyond Chocolate: How to Stop Yo-Yo Dieting and Lose Weight For Good,* was published in 2006, it was the first time the British public had been introduced to the idea of intuitive eating in an approachable and practical format. At the time, we were considered radical and even revolutionary. Up to then, women had two options: 1) they could buy into the myth of rapid and easy weight-loss sold by the dieting industry, or 2) they had to just grin and bear it and join the 'fat and happy' camp. With *Beyond Chocolate,* we offered them the third way – that by having a balanced, healthy relationship with food and our bodies, weight-loss is simply a welcome byproduct.

Today, we are delighted to see this idea becoming more and more mainstream! Thanks to the tireless work of women like Julie who have drawn on their personal experience and professional skills to support a growing number of people taking the leap and going down a different path. Julie helps you understand that FAT is not the issue, that it is merely a symptom. FAT is indeed not a four-letter word.

Julie's inspirational, no-nonsense and extremely practical Daily Lessons are clearly rooted in scientific knowledge. But here is a nutritionist with a very special twist. Rather than simply laying out an eating plan and expecting readers to follow blindly, she combines her understating of both the body and *the mind*. She knows that the key is to show people *how* to make changes, and *how* to motivate themselves to overcome unhelpful habits of a lifetime. She does this with a kindness, compassion and empathy that is truly rare.

Change is often difficult. Many of us resist it for one reason or another. Julie understands this so well. With this in mind she guides her readers to take tiny steps, to make small changes, which as you see, will have a BIG impact. We have seen how crucial this method is for long-term, sustainable weight loss. Anyone can alter the way they eat by going on a diet for a few weeks or even months. But the changes are fleeting and temporary. Without taking a close look at our habitual patterns, and transforming our limited thinking, eventually we'll revert back to what we know.

Julie's Daily Lessons make it possible to experiment with new concepts and learn new behaviors so that there's no going back. The process is kind, gentle and profoundly empowering. When we make a choice to look after ourselves rather than push and punish ourselves into a new regime, success is guaranteed. Change comes naturally and easily.

When we gave up dieting, over ten years ago, and decided to transform the way we approached weight loss, we made a commitment to ourselves to **take action.** Reading books and having good intentions is not enough. There can be no change without commitment and action. We cannot think of a better teacher than Julie Hammerstein to inspire you to make that commitment to yourself. We know you will enjoy reading this book and trust that you will put each lesson into practice… therein lies the freedom.

Sophie and Audrey Boss
The Chocolate Fairies
London 1 October 2010

CONTENTS

ACKNOWLEDGEMENTS

I am blessed to have extraordinary people in my life, whom I can now thank publicly.

It is with deep gratitude that I thank my coach, Lisa Jimenez. This book would have been long in the waiting without her encouragement, guidance, love, strength, compassion, and expertise. The day I met Lisa, I knew a profound shift was happening in my life. I was ready for massive change, and my prayers were answered when I heard Lisa on a radio interview the morning of my 41st birthday. I immediately signed up for her Mastermind coaching program, which has been the single best investment I've made in my business and my life. Lisa showed me how to create my world... that if I want greatness, to envision and live into greatness. If I want love, to envision and live into love. If I want to transform the Fat Kid Mentality, end the suffering, and eradicate obesity, to write this book. Lisa has a gift for moving people into action through her words, and I am honored to have her as my writing coach and partner in this book. "Thank you, Lisa, for helping manifest peace, prosperity, and global change!"

And to my editor, Vicki McCown, whom we endearingly refer to as "Picky Vicki." I had total confidence in her craft and learned valuable writing lessons from her excellent skill. I appreciate her patience and clarity and am so thankful to have her on my team.

To my joy and inspiration, Max. What a privilege to be his mommy and share this journey with such a wise and special soul. He teaches me that life is fun, and that health is our birthright. "I love you, honey." And to his father and my former husband, Grant Barnhill, who paid for the nutrition schooling that changed my career path fifteen years ago.

Thank you to my soul-mate Andrew, who is my soft place to land, cooking me fabulous meals, rubbing my feet, and providing the perfect respite with his love and unending support. He moved me into action when I felt doubt and uncertainty, reminding me that someone who expects greatness has a different "normal" than most. "I LOVE YOU.".

Unending appreciation to my parents, Ann, Clark, Bill and Marcy. Many of my actions and beliefs are deeply rooted in their teachings and I am so grateful for these lessons.

A special appreciation goes to my gorgeous mother Ann, who serves as my role model and guiding light. Words cannot express my gratitude for EVERYTHING she does – helping me with errands, caring for Max, and showing me unconditional love and respect at every step. "You are a saint!".

Such gratitude for my siblings, nieces, and nephews – Clay, Rebecca, Peyton, Hunter, Kyle, Blake, Michelle, John, Alex, Diana, AJ, Emily, Walker, Joey, TJ, Lauren, Kelly, and Wes – who bring me immense joy, laughter, and love.

So many wonderful friends bless me every day with their support, kindness, and acceptance. A special thank you to Shelley McClellan, who has been my unwavering support and "soul sister", and the person I count on for advice or a bellyaching laugh.

Contributions from my dear friends, Theresa Byrne and Chelsea Frankel, who shared their insight in a couple of the chapters, and whom I trust explicitly in their loving wishes for this book.

Thank you to the numerous clients, customers, and colleagues who allow me to do my work and help me to spread my message. They are the catalysts for change, and I truly appreciate their confidence in my care.

When I wake every morning, I thank God and my spiritual guides for showing me that all is well and perfect. I am in service and living with purpose. Thank you for this glorious journey called My Life. And thank you for calling me out so that this book can truly serve others and transform lives.

INTRODUCTION

I spent half my life feeling bad about being fat.

Not only did I feel bad, I believed I *was* bad.

And all the messages around me confirmed that being thin was good and being fat was bad.

So as an impressionable child with a chubby belly and a propensity for fast food and sugar, I formed the idea early on that I was the Fat Kid in the "bad" category.

This was affirmed whenever someone called me "fat." Possibly a boy on the playground, a jealous friend, or an angry sibling – it was as if someone pulled the worst word out of the dictionary and threw it at me like a dagger.

From the time I was nine years old, up until my thirty-third birthday, I lived in daily torment about the shape of my body.

Every mirror I passed, I would hear the resounding message:

"You are fat, fat, fat!"

It never failed.

I was convinced I was the Fat Kid forever.

Yet, here's what's so interesting.

For ten of those years I thought I was the Fat Kid, I was actually thin!

That's right. At age twenty-three I weighed a healthy 118 pounds. I controlled my calories and I ran every day so as not to feel guilty.

But it didn't matter. This really had no bearing on how I felt every time I looked in the mirror.

You know why?

Because even after changing my life and getting to a healthy weight, I still lived in a Fat Kid's body. And when you live in a Fat Kid's body, you think with a Fat Kid's mind.

And that's why I wrote this book.

When I first started as a professional nutritionist, I noticed patterns about myself, and my clients, that were keeping us stuck in old ways of eating. I realized, that until we dealt with what I call our "Fat Kid Mentality," we'll always be unhappy with our weight, and we'll forever battle with our ideas around food.

Here's a perfect example:

Notice in the paragraph above where I said that I controlled my calories and exercised every day so as not to feel guilty. Sounds like a decent approach. But notice the subtle implication of this. Unless I controlled my calories and ran every day, I was going to feel guilty. Can you relate to this? Are you thinking, "Yes, I always feel guilty too?"

If so, then I'm glad you are reading the book.

Because that is how a Fat Kid thinks!

A Fat Kid believes that food is to be CONTROLLED, and if she can't control it she's failed. When a Fat Kid fails, she feels GUILT, so she'll do anything to make sure she doesn't fail.

So despite my healthy weight and habits, I had no freedom until I transformed my Fat Kid Mentality. I was still controlled by the mindset of being a Fat Kid.

Before we go on, let me back up a bit and tell you my story.

Let's just say that as a kid I was chubby. I wasn't obese, but you could see I had a belly and more fat than my friends.

Trust me, there was enough fat for the boys to call me fat. There was enough fat for my parents to feel concern. There was enough fat to make me pay close attention to what society deemed as "being fat." I was constantly comparing myself to skinny friends, girls on the beach, or the standards on TV and in teen magazines.

This made me unhappy.

Actually, it made me hate myself.

My self-loathing perpetuated my infatuation with food, and my infatuation with food perpetuated my self-loathing. **The more**

self-hate, the more I ate. Did I know this then? Of course not, I was a kid!

So I continued to eat candy, sweets, and fast food.

I knew this wasn't good for me, but I found incredible comfort in sugar and starch. I would come home from school and eat half a sleeve of cookies, then go back for a handful of greasy chips, then dinner, then seconds, then dessert.

My parents knew my dietary habits were no good. Yet they didn't want to make a big deal out of my weight. Like many parents, they didn't want me to have a complex around food.

Then one day someone made a comment about my fat butt. So I put myself on a diet.

I was thirteen years old.

I'll never forget one of my dinner plans that included liver. Gross! Then I did a diet that called for 500 calories a day and shots in my butt administered by a nurse at a weight loss clinic. Ouch! One summer all I ate was hard-boiled egg whites, cooked asparagus, and watermelon. Wow, did I lose weight.

Do you think I kept if off?

Nope. I cycled through diets every six months, and by the time I was nineteen years old, I was fifty pounds overweight and super unhappy. Since starting that first diet as a young teen, I had gotten fatter and fatter every year.

You know why I couldn't keep it off?

Because I still **BELIEVED I was a Fat Kid!** And when you feel like a Fat Kid, you'll **THINK** and **BEHAVE** like a Fat Kid.

Do you think a Fat Kid knows when to turn off the Fat Kid thoughts?

He doesn't unless someone shows him how. And in all my efforts toward weight loss, no one ever told me I could actually shift my way of thinking.

Instead, the lessons and diet plans were all about calorie CONTROL and avoiding GUILT!

Which is why I failed. Because this way of thinking is the Fat Kid Mentality!

This way of thinking says that being fat is bad. It's a mindset that sets up negative beliefs around food, weight, and what it means to be healthy. It's a way of Being that our society supports with all the messages around good food versus bad food, good habits versus bad habits, perfect bodies versus ugly bodies.

So whether you're fat, thin, tall, short, young, or old, YOU have the Fat Kid Mentality too. If you don't believe me, then please take a moment to complete this questionnaire:

1) Do you have a hard time saying the word "fat" to describe someone who is overweight?
2) When you call someone "fat," do you feel judgment, criticism, or disgust?
3) Do you think people who are thin are better than people who are fat?
4) Do you judge yourself, whether good or bad, by the types and amounts of food you eat?
5) Do you judge others, whether good or bad, by the types and amounts of food they eat?

6) Do you have conversations with yourself every time you eat? (Really consider this one…what did you think this morning when you skipped breakfast? What did you tell yourself when you had that glass of wine last night, the dessert, or the burger? Did you think you were being good when you chose the salad instead of the bread?).

7) Do you count calories?

8) Do you disregard calories yet have conversations with yourself about portion sizes?

9) Do you justify your food choices? (e.g. – "I'm eating this because I deserve it!")

10) Do you praise your food choices? (e.g. – "I would never eat junk food!")

11) Are you worried your children will mimic your eating habits?

12) Do you boast when you or your children eat their vegetables?

13) Is dieting something you consider good or bad?

14) Are there foods you avoid because when you eat them you feel guilty?

15) Are you having negative thoughts about this questionnaire?

If you answered yes to just **one** of these questions, then you have the Fat Kid Mentality. But don't worry, you're not alone. Most people have this mentality, which sets you up for limiting thoughts and beliefs around food that keep you trapped.

Question #1 is the impetus for writing this book. It is also what birthed the title **FAT Is Not Four-Letter Word.** In addressing and eradicating our Fat Kid Mentality, we erase the belief that being fat makes you bad.

I am here to finally pull out the daggers – the words, the beliefs, and the images – that injure you and keep you stuck in the Fat Kid Mentality!

It's not just you.

It's society. It's a cultural mindset that says FAT is bad, food is to be CONTROLLED, and when you FAIL, you should feel GUILTY.

By reading this book you will break through this way of thinking forever. And when you finally transform your Fat Kid Mentality, you will achieve a healthy weight, have freedom around food, and never worry about being fat again.

Here's the rest of my story.

At nineteen, I realized I was tired of dieting. I was tired of trying things that people said would work and then failing. I was tired of being stuck in my story of "I'm the Fat Kid."

So here's what I did.

I started running. The first day I went eight blocks. That's it, just eight blocks. Sound like nothing?

By the end of the year I was running six miles.

And here's what happened next:

1) I cut out fast food and sugar.
2) I quit unhealthy habits like smoking and drinking too much alcohol.
3) I found that running alleviated my stress and boosted my mood.
4) I got good grades and landed a great job right after college.

Finally, I started to see that I could be something other than fat. I really began to think and live like a healthy person!

But my work wasn't over. As said above, I still had the thought patterns that kept me stuck in the Fat Kid way of thinking. I was able to maintain healthy weight, but it was maintained through CONTROL and GUILT.

I didn't come to my self-realization about the Fat Kid Mentality until later in life. It became clear to me after several years of healing my own issues around weight, and then coaching thousands of clients to heal theirs, that everyone has some sort of limiting belief around food that started in childhood. These beliefs support the feelings around food such as guilt, control, fear, and limitation.

You see, your current habits around food and exercise didn't just happen overnight. In reality, you've had these ideas around food your entire life. Because even if you were the thin kid, there were still images and patterns that were set up by society that said,

"FAT is bad."

As a result, you set up limiting beliefs around food and exercise that kept you from being FAT and BAD.

And if you were the Fat Kid, then your patterns were just reinforced by the societal messages that said,

"**YOU** are bad."

Do you see the trap?

Do you see how we ALL must shift our mindset if we are going to create true change and eradicate obesity?

If we **THINK** like Fat Kids, then we'll **BEHAVE** like Fat Kids, and we'll raise a nation of Fat Kids.

So if you're blaming yourself for lack of willpower, stop it! And notice...

THAT's the Fat Kid Mentality.

If you feel you have no control over your cravings, stop it! And notice...

THAT's the Fat Kid Mentality.

If you think living healthy comes only through guilt, stop it! And notice...

THAT's the Fat Kid Mentality.

This book is all about getting you to notice your Fat Kid Mentality. If you keep listening to the current messages of the Fat Kid Mentality, you will continue to enforce them. Remember, when you THINK you're the Fat Kid, you will ACT like the Fat Kid.

So what relevance does this have for you?

By reading this book, you'll find out. You will understand why I've made it my life's mission to eradicate obesity by transforming the Fat Kid Mentality in all of us.

I am here to help you realize that achieving a healthy weight isn't difficult, and, most importantly, it is your birthright to be happy, fit, and whole.

My philosophy is this: **Small Change, Big Impact.**™

To transform the Fat Kid Mentality, you can't expect to overhaul your life in one day.

Six miles my first day out? That seemed impossible. Eight blocks? Look what THAT did.

By committing to small, intentional changes every day, you will move away from the Fat Kid Mentality and create the results that set you free from this way of thinking for life.

This book is about the small steps. It's about taking on what you can at the time and celebrating every victory that gets you closer to your gifts. Some of the biggest victories happen when you recognize that the little things matter.

Like eight blocks.

This book is also interactive, so I'm asking for your full participation.

The Daily Lesson chapters are set up to teach an overarching lesson, followed by a **Small Change** action step. Some action steps will require that you write in a journal or spaces provided on the page. Or I may ask you to change your morning schedule, or alter your daily meals. You will also be challenged to close your eyes and imagine, spend time in gratitude, or have a conversation with a loved one.

These action steps are all designed to put you in the experience of the Small Change, so that you can manifest the results immediately.

In the last section of each Daily Lesson chapter, I will share **Big Impact** stories from my life and the lives of my clients – people who have made tremendous shifts in their health by implementing the Small Changes discussed.

By following the steps and fully diving into the Fourteen Daily Lessons, you'll start to retrain your brain and radically reverse physiology towards better health. You'll be set free from the Fat Kid Mentality and no longer have it rule your life. You'll walk away from dieting and stop forcing something that is not in synch with your true nature.

Only with a radical transformation in your thoughts, beliefs, and relationship with food and exercise can you break through the Fat Kid Mentality and realize a whole new healthy you.

Thank you for letting me be your guide. I look forward to our journey.

Warmly,

Julie

Chapter One
END TRIBAL THINKING

I t's a fact. Human beings need to feel loved and accepted. This basic need inspires us to join groups, build friendships, and even get married.

According to Maslow's Hierarchy of Needs, this belonging falls just behind our most basic needs for food, shelter, and water. And since most of us don't worry about where our next meal is coming from, we have the freedom to foster relationships and develop social standing.

And this is where the trouble begins.

The need to belong is so strong in our society that it creates a tribal way of thinking that makes you fat.

Let me first explain the power of tribal thinking.

To be part of something bigger than yourself is not a contemporary phenomenon. Humans have always formed groups – or tribes – as a means for survival. Our ancestors formed tribes as a way to successfully hunt for food, build adequate shelter, and to protect each other from predators.

Tribes – or societies – were skillfully designed with common principles and belief systems to ensure harmony. In our earliest existence, tribes were created for the survival of the community. Survival relied on conformity, and those who botched the system posed a big threat to the group. It makes sense that tribal thinking was useful and necessary.

Yet, where this was once needed for survival, in today's world, certain forms of tribal thinking are killing you!

Why? Because when you look at the tribal thinking around health and wellness, you are conforming to a value system that is broken.

When tribal thinking, or the need to belong, causes you to sacrifice your self-care or self-respect to fit in or impress others, you are basing your personal value on factors outside yourself.

This is so dangerous.

Rather than valuing who you are, society places more importance on what you do, what you look like, and what you have.

If you have an innate need to be valued, and believe that value comes through material possessions, how will this shape your behavior? Would you work long hours to get a raise? Would you allow this to take precedence over things like exercise or eating a healthy lunch?

You better believe you would! Remember, this need for acceptance is an insatiable need. Gone unchecked, it starts to rule your life and your habits, so that you become unaware of your body's inherent needs.

So, what about you?

Are you more afraid of not belonging than you are of the sacrifices you must make to belong? Are you wiling to risk your health – your life – to commit to the material things that make you feel loved and accepted? If so, then you are a victim of tribal thinking.

As you desperately seek to belong – sometimes with the intensity of life or death – you are ignoring the one thing that truly sustains life…your health.

Societies are formed on this very premise. Industries are built to support the hardworking individual just trying to get ahead. It is very easy to conform to a ten-hour workday when you know you can pick up a fast food meal. Or take a drug if you get diseased from being sedentary. Or sit your kids in front of the TV when you don't have time to play with them outside.

This is tribal thinking.

Consider the media. Every day you are exposed to images that reinforce personal value in what you have, "You will be more desirable if you own this car." "You will have more friends if you live in this neighborhood."

This is tribal thinking.

But it doesn't stop with value attached to wealth. There are other cultural norms that support the need to belong. "You will be happy if you are thin." "You will be more desirable if you fit into these jeans."

Wow – can you see the trap of tribal thinking? It's insatiable. It's automatic. It's a reflex. And it dictates every decision and every aspect of your life.

This becomes more confusing when you consider the opposing forces of tribal thinking.

You are told to work out, so there's a health club on every corner. Yet next to the clubs are the fast food restaurants that support the quick meal while driving to the next meeting, soccer game, or after-school event.

You enroll your kids in sports so they can have fun and "fit in" with their friends. Yet with the intense schedule of all the soccer games, comes the necessity to forgo precious family time over dinner.

You are told that to get hired by a good company you must be a well-rounded person. Yet once you are hired, you have no time for all the things that made you hirable – hobbies, family, sports, and self-care.

Tribal thinking has caused most Americans to over-schedule their lives in a way thatcompromises their health. So much so that we've come to rely on diet pills and quick-fix measures where a trip to the grocery store means picking up a frozen pizza and a box of Slim Fast.

You CAN do it differently.

I am not discounting your right to live a life of abundance and prosperity. I wholeheartedly support people who are intimately connected to their vision and are doing what it takes to live in prosperity. I'm one of them!

The difference lies in the motivation. If you believe you will be loved because you are thin and rich, then you are a victim of tribal thinking. And this thinking further enforces the Fat Kid Mentality that says, "I'll do whatever it takes to be accepted."

So here's your challenge. Only when you KNOW personal value based on self-love and integrity are you able to break the social norms and erase your Fat Kid Mentality.

By placing more value on the joy and happiness that resides within, you can easily discern how you want to spend your time and where YOU want to place value.

This won't happen overnight, trust me. It takes a total paradigm shift to move away from the tribal thinking and allow your intuition to guide you.

Imagine this: You're standing in the middle of a tightly packed crowd. The crowd is anxious and fighting for space. You peer above the crowd, and outside the circle is a huge open space. There is sunlight and the freedom to swing your arms and breathe deeply. The space bubbles with joy!

Now just stick one toe into that open space. Just one toe. Then a leg and an arm. Then half your body. How do you think you'd feel if half your body was entrenched in the crowd and the other was flowing freely in the open space? Which one do you think is more desirable – chaos or freedom?

I bet you'll choose freedom.

Freedom is what happens when your actions are based on what you know to be true for yourself. It is then that you are truly choosing your outcomes. You start to honor what feels right for YOU. You walk in unwavering conviction that you will get the results you desire.

For example. When I decided to start running in college, it meant I had to step outside the realm of what all of my friends were doing. Rather than hanging out in the sun all afternoon and partying at night, I had to be the odd man out and go for my run every day.

I didn't want to go out every night, because I wouldn't get my run in the next day. I didn't want to hang out every afternoon, because I needed to stay on schedule if I was going to stay committed. So, I risked being seen as rigid or boring and not fitting in.

For a while my friends suggested they were sad because I'd changed and wasn't hanging out with them. As soon as my friends noticed I was different, I could have chosen to stop running to secure my place in the tribe.

But I stood in my truth. I held firm to the belief that exercising was the key to creating a better life.

And you know what?

When I started to lose weight, their opinions changed. When I got straight A's and secured a summer internship with a reputable marketing firm, their opinions changed.

Soon, my friends joined me. They went for runs with me. They joined me at the law library for study time. They quit unhealthy habits like smoking and eating fast food. They began moving into their own greatness, and we started to create new paradigms for our group.

Now, consider this happening for you. YOU can show the people around you the incredible payoffs of tapping into their innate desires and doing it differently.

When you choose to live based on what OTHERS want for you, you set yourself up to fail. Your actions are derived from something outside yourself, and when you don't succeed, you blame others. "This diet doesn't work." "My boss is a jerk." "My husband doesn't support me." "My life is out of control."

This mindset keeps you trapped! And honestly, how does it feel to always point the finger? Do you feel empowered? Do you feel joyful and content? Do you feel love towards yourself when you defiantly take a stand against others?

I bet not. That's not freedom. That's entrapment.

What you are seeking cannot be satisfied until you have given it to yourself.

You know what that is?

Love.

People who love themselves do not treat themselves poorly. They do not sabotage their efforts. They do not let others determine their future.

And the best part, when you love yourself, you act in loving ways.

When you identify what's truly important to you, you will be amazed at how QUICKLY you can accomplish your goals. You will no longer feel threatened. No one can defeat you, because your self-love is stronger than any criticism or voice of doubt.

That is the freedom I refer to when you live "outside the circle."

It may seem scary at first, because we are programmed to believe that there is safety in crowds. Yet, when I realized I loved myself too much to treat my body poorly, my whole life turned around.

So you might be asking, "How do I learn to love myself?"

I did a lot of introspection. I know it's my birthright to have a healthy and perfectly functioning body.

So I say this to you: It is YOUR BIRTHRIGHT AND YOUR NATURAL STATE to have a healthy and perfectly functioning body!

When you realize this, you will see that what you want you already have! You just need to uncover your perfect self – it's right there under the surface of fear, self-doubt, and the Fat Kid Mentality that says, "You can't have this."

So for you, finding self-love might be reading this book. Or possibly it's reading other powerful books or listening to CDs. Maybe it's working with a therapist. It might be sitting in meditation every morning or getting in touch with nature. It could be journaling or taking a vacation.

Here's what it feels like. When you feel the calm that follows silence...that is self-love. When you feel confident as you play the piano or sing to the radio...that is self-love. When you feel compassion towards others or take a stand for a cause...that is self-love.

When you listen to your body and stop basing your value on what others think...you guessed it, self-love.

Once you recognize this and see it as something extraordinary and not just a passing thought or feeling, then you are ready to take the next steps in breaking your Fat Kid Mentality.

You can start small. You can stick your toe out with small changes. And these small changes will cause a big impact by moving you into a natural state of self-love and total conviction that optimal health is yours.

In your tangible world, you will need some ideas. You can feel self-love, but what can you actually do to break tribal thinking and make a difference in your life?

Here are some examples:

1) Leave work thirty minutes early to take a walk with your kids.
2) Wake up twenty minutes early to powerfully send your kids into the world with a healthy breakfast, rather than a bowl of sugary cereal.
3) Say no to the chips that come with your lunch and choose the apple.
4) Prepare healthy snacks on Sunday for the soccer games during the week.
5) Skip the latte and fuel your body with meditation for that afternoon lull!
6) Say no to the cocktail and choose water.
7) Decide that a fit, healthy body will get you the promotion at work.
8) Skip dessert and explain to your hosts that you are trying to set a good example for your family.
9) Have a discussion with your spouse about how you can each fit in twenty minutes of exercise tomorrow.
10) Refrain from gossip and look for ways to support others.

Just stick a toe outside the circle for right now. Which example do you choose? Write down which small effort, from this list or your own, you are willing to commit to this week:

_____

_____

The biggest shift you'll have to make is with your values. Where do you place value?

Is it on the perceived acceptance you get from others when you "fit in"? Or do you place more value on being healthy, happy, and immune from obesity and disease?

Once you make this decision, the rest just follows the lessons spelled out in this book.

In the next chapter I'll shatter the myth about willpower and dieting and explore what it really takes to break through your Fat Kid Mentality to be fit and healthy for life.

Chapter Two
DIET, WILLPOWER, AND DENIAL

U nless you've been meditating in a cave for the past forty years, you recognize the words "diet" and "willpower." Right?

Isn't the "right diet" what you've been searching for? If you could just find it, you would lose the weight. And if you had more "willpower" to follow the right diet... then you would be fit! And, if diet and willpower continue to be evasive, there's always denial. If you don't admit there's a problem, it will go away.

Sound familiar?

These words and the beliefs they generate are a myth. And the myth is deadly. In fact, these three words – diet, willpower, and denial – and the power they hold are actually perpetuating your Fat Kid Mentality, and the world's health crisis of obesity.

And this is no longer tolerable.

Please allow me to bust the weight-loss myths and present you with the facts; facts will free you from your unwinnable battle with weight and set you up for victory. You will change the way you live, because you will truly crave all that is good for you. **Healthy living will become who you are, not just what you do.**

This book is about a total transformation of your mindset and your being. And this process of transformation begins with exposing the myths that are keeping you bound in old patterns.

Myth #1: If I could just find the "right" diet...

How many diets have you tried? Ten? Five? Two?

Even if it's only one, you are reading this book so it must not have made a lasting impression.

That's because diets don't work.

Here's why.

FACT: Dieting keeps you stuck in the cycle of dieting.

What is the difference between diet and dieting? Do you know? When you get this distinction, you are free to create a whole new way of being around food and exercise.

Here's the distinction:

Dieting is something you do for a segment of time or until you achieve your desired result, whereas **Diet** is a sustainable pattern of living that exists every day and lasts for the rest of your life.

You've heard the statement "Diets don't work." This is partially true, but only in your understanding of it. In this phrase, the word "diet" represents a plan designed to make you lose weight.

But it's not that diets don't work. A sound DIET does work. It's DIETING that doesn't work. Do you hear the difference?

Think of it this way:

Diet = Long-term pattern (Lifestyle) **Dieting** = Short-term deprivation (Quick fix).

The difference is that "dieting" assumes you do it once, and then you stop. Just consider what you are creating in your mindset when you read the following definition:

Dieting: The practice of eating (and drinking) in a regulated fashion to achieve a particular, short-term objective.

The operative phrase is "short-term." What's implied here is that once you're "there," and have achieved your desired weight, you can go back to your normal, unregulated ways of eating.

The other distinction I want you to see is that dieting sets you up to believe that it has to be HARD. For a short period of time, you have to tough it out, and then you're done.

And when something is hard, what do you need more of?

WILLPOWER!

Which leads us to...

Myth #2: If I just had more willpower...

Can you relate? Every person I've consulted as a nutritionist has said those words.

And guess what? It's a lie! In fact, "If I just had more willpower" is the very belief that will ensure you stay fat.

Every time you are dieting, you create a pattern. I call it the "Dieting Dance." You know the steps. You know them so well you don't even have to think about them anymore. You can do the Dieting Dance blindfolded.

Here's a description of **The Dieting Dance:**

Search for a great diet. Find it. Have enough willpower to just do it until you get the weight off. The weight comes off. You celebrate! Life is good. You go back to your old habitual way of eating now that you are not dieting. Weight comes back on. Life is hard. You are unhappy. So you...

Search for the next great diet (because obviously the last one was flawed.) Find it. Have enough willpower to just do it until you get the weight off. The weight comes off. You celebrate! Life is good. You go back to your old habitual patterns of eating now that you are not dieting. Weight comes back on. Life is hard. You are unhappy. So you...

Search for the next great diet (because obviously the last one was flawed.) Find it. Have enough willpower to just do it until you get the weight off. The weight comes off. You celebrate! Life is good. You go back to your old habitual patterns of eating now that you are not dieting. Weight comes back on. Life is hard. You are unhappy. So you...

...keep doing the dance.

When you get caught up in the myth of willpower, you find yourself going to extremes. You are stuck in a constant pattern of win or lose, because you have relinquished all control.

When you think about it, you are like everyone else who's living out the Dieting Dance. Yet, you feel like you are special, like you're the only one doing the dance.

But here's what will truly differentiate you and set you free.

FACT: Losing weight has nothing to do with willpower but more to do with reasoning.

You and I have equal gifts. Yes, we are special and unique in many ways, but we all share certain qualities of the mind. We can discern, for example, the difference between hot and cold. On a more intellectual level, we have the inherent ability to discern what supports our well-being and what does not.

These gifts are called "intellectual factors." Now when I say they are inherent, that means they are already within us. We are born with them.

Your job is to be aware of these God-given intellectual factors and develop them. When you tap into these intellectual factors, you will powerfully transform your life and successfully create a healthy and fit body.

Here are the Six Intellectual Factors that give you the power to change old patterns and create healthier responses to food, exercise, and healthy habits:

1. Reason

Your mind gives you the ability to receive and process information. It does this through your five senses: sight, smell, taste, hearing, and touch.

When information comes in through one of these five senses, you have a programmed response.

These responses happen automatically, because they come from the subconscious mind. For example, you see a ring of fire from the burner on a stove. Your programmed response is: "Fire is hot, don't touch it."

I know it sounds really simple and obvious, but this is your subconscious mind making the decision for you: "Don't touch the fire!"

Now this information – fire is hot – was introduced to your senses through touch at some point in your life. When you felt the hot fire, you decided not to touch fire again because it hurts.

Here's the reality. You can TRAIN your subconscious mind to have the same response to unhealthy habits.

Let's use eating a doughnut as an example. You see the doughnut and your programmed response is to eat it because it tastes good. This is your TRIGGERED response and habitual pattern that is ingrained in your subconscious mind.

Now, what I want you to get is that this triggered response to the doughnut was created by you. And you have the power to shift the subconscious, triggered response any time you want. Saying the same thing in another way, when you use your intellectual factor of reasoning to create a new pattern in your brain for the doughnut, you actually create a new triggered response that will pop up subconsciously and automatically – without effort!

If you take the time to realize how the programmed response of eating the doughnut is not serving you, you can reprogram the response. You can RETRAIN the brain to see the doughnut and be reminded of how it makes you feel depressed, tired, and bloated.

Do you see the power you have? You can create a different scenario for your subconscious to follow, which then becomes JUST AS AUTOMATIC as not touching the hot fire.

Eat the doughnut, feel depressed. Touch the fire, get burned.

It's all in how you use your five senses to reprogram responses that create better outcomes. You have this choice.

The new response? Don't eat the doughnut.

2. Imagination

This is the most powerful of the intellectual factors because you can create anything you want just by imagining it. That's not to say that action steps don't need to follow. But once the thought is there, you can put your desires into motion. Imagination gives you the framework and the starting point for better possibilities with better outcomes.

It's no mistake that when you imagine something you want, you begin seeing that "something" everywhere you go. You see the car you've imagined driving. You want a vacation and find travel brochures randomly placed in coffee shops. You want a new home and start noticing more for sale signs on your way to work.

Imagination is the portal to reality.

Picture yourself fit, healthy, happy, and beautiful. What would that look like? How would that make you feel? There's no right or wrong answer here...just imagine what that would mean for you.

The best way to open up to your stream of imagination is to get laser-focused on what you want. Once you know what that is, you will actually train yourself to notice the little clues that get you closer to your dreams.

Imagination creates awareness to new opportunities.

If you never imagine driving the nice car, then it is not part of your thought process. As soon as it's in your thoughts – or your imagination – you will naturally start looking at ways to get the car.

It is the same with your health.

If you've never imagined having a toned body, then your brain does not have the right information to work with. All it has is the information you've given it – a flabby and sluggish body.

When you do imagine a toned body, you are giving your sub-conscious NEW marching orders to create a toned body. All of a sudden the brain has the vision to ATTRACT a healthy and toned body into your realm of possibility. It's like giving your brain the paint-by-numbers to create a new you.

Here's an example:

For years you've been imagining healthy food will taste bland and boring. Your brain sends the signal "There's no reason to try this."

Instead, imagine eating fresh, healthy foods from the Farmer's Market every weekend. If you imagine this food will taste delicious and make you feel amazing, then your brain will send the signal "Buy fresh food." Your imagination transforms your thoughts and your thoughts trigger the brain automatically to say, "Hmmm... healthy food is yummy!"

Now you know how much power you have in using your imag-ination to transform your thoughts and your habitual brain triggers.

Isn't this amazing?

You are born with the ability to use your imagination to your advantage! It's not just creating a bunch of pipe dreams or false hopes. It's creating exactly what you want in life and giving your subconscious the visual to put your dreams into action.

3. Memory

You have a perfect memory. Unless there is a structural or chemical imbalance, you have the capacity to recall information in a very efficient manner.

You've heard people say, "I never remember people's names" or "I can never remember a good joke." It's not that their memory is bad, it's that they haven't trained or exercised their memory to tap into the information that is stored there.

In the game of health, YOU have the power to use your memory for good and empowering visions. Recall memories around food and wellbeing that made you happy, gave you power, and brought you joy. Remember how ALIVE you felt the last time you went on a hike in the woods or ate a fresh, juicy peach.

Equally, you can remember the last time you ate three pieces of greasy cheese pizza. Remember how good the first few bites tasted? Now, remember how the second and third pieces tasted. Even though they had the same ingredients as the first piece, the sensation was very different after the first few bites.

This is no accident.

This is your body telling you that the first few bites are all you need. After that, you will just feel stuffed and uncomfortable, wishing you hadn't eaten three pieces. This is your mind and body's intelligence saying, "Remember how you felt the last time you did this?"

Memory is the portal to foresight.

I get my clients to use their memory before they make a decision around food and exercise.

For example, I had a client who was trying to quit drinking wine at night. Before she poured her first glass, I had her stop and remember what she felt like that morning when she had woken up foggy and tired for work.

This recollection gave her the foresight to choose a different outcome for the next day. What she really wanted was to wake up, go for a walk, and get a healthy start. She is reminded daily how amazing she feels when she does this, so now she makes different choices and opts out of the wine.

That's the power of memory!

You have this Intellectual Factor in you. Use your memory to trigger positive and empowering actions towards food and exercise. Soon these actions will become so much a part of who you are that you will do them without thinking. You are getting the subconscious to work for you by making healthier choices with ease.

4. Perception

This gives you the ability to look at any situation from a different point of view. The beauty in this is that you are free to perceive a situation any way you choose. You can wake up every morning and DECIDE how you want to view your day.

The healthiest people are the ones who wake up every day and feel excited to exercise and eat a fresh, healthy breakfast. If you think these habits are too hard or tedious, this is just your perception. Healthy people perceive them differently.

It's like waking up on a sunny day and deciding to feel great. Then on a rainy day you decide to feel horrible. Your perception is that the rainy day is bad and the sunny day is good. What if you chose to be happy and grateful despite your surroundings?

The other day I went to a funeral. I could have decided to be depressed. Instead I chose to be thankful that I was alive to enjoy the day and to celebrate my friend's life in the way she would have wanted.

It comes down to a simple choice.

Do you perceive health as too difficult and unattainable? If so, it will be. Or, do you perceive health as essential, exciting, and something to look forward to every day? If so, it will be.

I was working with a client who hated exercise. Actually, what she really hated was sweating, which she found "gross" and "inconvenient."

I actually love to sweat. I think sweating is sexy, and it cleans out all the yucky stuff that our bodies have to deal with every day.

I asked my client to shift her thinking and perceive sweat as the very thing that would cure her Type II diabetes. We didn't even work on diet for a few weeks. I just asked her to make a list of "Twenty Good Things About Sweat."

She did it.

As she put her list together, she decided that sweating could possibly make her skin healthier. She also chose to believe that if she wasn't so afraid to sweat that she could enroll in a hot yoga class where she would meet new people. And once she saw what the yoga could lead to, like fitting into her bikini, she decided to change her thinking about sweating and started to turn her life around.

She enrolled in the yoga class where she met a man who is now her boyfriend. She lost weight and controls her diabetes without medication.

It's all in how you decide to see a situation. When you choose to see a situation in a positive light, with healthy outcomes, you train your subconscious to automatically see things working for you, rather than against you.

5. Intuition

This factor gives you the ability to pick up vibrations (feelings) about your surroundings. It gives you a "knowing" about people and situations around you. When you are intuitive, or aware, you can sense certain things about your surroundings that will aid in your response.

The idea is to use your intuition for positive results.

When you experience a gut feeling, this is your intuition speaking to you. It is your direct connection to the intelligence within you.

For example, have you ever sensed that a friend is in need or that something is bothering a family member, but you haven't had a direct conversation with that person about a specific problem? Still, because that inner feeling is so strong, you pick up the phone just to check in. Or maybe you meet someone and your intuition immediately tells you, "He is a good person and can be trusted."

You can use this same intuition for the betterment of your mind and body.

Let's say you've never been told that sugar gives you a headache. No doctor has diagnosed this, but every time you eat something sweet you get a headache. Sometimes even the thought of eating something sweet can bring on the hint of a headache.

This thought is your intuition! It's like an old, wise soul saying, "This is what's happening here, please pay attention."

You have a choice: to trust your intuition and respond in a way that creates better outcomes or choose to ignore your intuition and pay the consequences.

Try applying this to the type of exercise you want to do.

I have a client who told me she doesn't like to run. She's tried it before, and she knows that it hurts her body and that it's not good for her knees. So I asked if there was another type of exercise that she might enjoy.

She said, "Something tells me that I'd really like cycling. I don't know what it is, but I just get a feeling that it would be good for my body, and that I'd really enjoy it."

That "something" was my client's intuition. On a deep level, she knew and trusted that cycling would be a good fit. To finish her story, she bought a bike, loves it, and continues to cycle about thirty to forty minutes every day.

So what am I trying to tell you?

I want you to understand that your intuition is telling you something about your current state of health. What is it saying? What is the loud message that you know to be true but are choosing not to listen to? Once you listen, you can move out of the negative behaviors or situations knowing you understand the absolute right thing to do.

6. Personal Will

Your will gives you the capability to focus energy on what you want and move forward with conviction. In developing this, you must first know what you want. Otherwise, you cannot willfully make decisions and choices that benefit your long- and short-term goals.

When you don't access personal will, you blame others when circumstances turn out differently than you'd hoped. But in reality, YOU are choosing that very experience. You are choosing to avoid a conversation with a friend. You are choosing to surround yourself with negative or positive people. You are choosing whether to exercise more or eat less.

I had a client I'd been coaching for about three years. Despite my efforts to transform his habitual patterns around food and get him to eat smaller portions, he just wasn't doing it. His weight would fluctuate annually, and when he didn't get the desired results, he would blame it on two things – his travel schedule and his wife.

One day I sat him down and asked, "Dave, why are you seeing me?"

He said, "To lose weight."

I responded, "Why do you want to lose weight?"

He was ready to jump in to his normal set of excuses, and then he stopped. He thought about it for a few moments then said humbly, "I want to be healthy. I also want to be a good role model for my family so that they don't have to suffer like I have."

I replied with tough love, "Then when are you going to stop making excuses?"

He sat there speechless. After a few seconds he just nodded his head. And that was it. I knew in that moment the shift had happened, and he was committed. He had tapped into the will, and there was no turning back.

In two weeks he came to my office and had lost two pounds. For the next thirty weeks he lost a pound a week for a total of thirty-two pounds. In the three years that he had been my client, he had never lost more than twelve pounds.

That is the power of will. That is what it means to CHOOSE your outcomes. When you have clarity around why you want to be fit, you tap into the power of will and find the conviction to stay committed to the daily steps that get the job done.

When you understand that you have the gift of choice, everything is graciously put in your hands to create whatever you want. It is your job then to move forward with conviction.

Your will is the portal to conviction.

I love that word – "conviction" – the way it sounds, what it means: "a strong persuasion or belief." I use this word daily when coaching my clients. When clients say, "I can't," "I always fail at this," "I repeat bad habits," I ask how much conviction – strong belief – is being given these negative statements.

Then I ask them to pay attention to how they feel when they think about a person they admire – a role model or a mentor. A profound shift takes place. They sit up straight, smile, and absolutely defend their belief in that person. They know, without a doubt, that this person will do the right thing and succeed.

Now I'll do this with you. We're going to shift to a belief in yourself. If you had conviction in your own potential, what would that create? How would you set yourself up for success, rather than perpetuate less desirable results?

You must willfully take on healthy habits to accomplish the truly grand. Will is what carries you when you think time will chip away at your dreams. It is what keeps you strong when negative people start to hack away at your plans. It is what creates the shift from doubtful thinking to the type of thinking that attracts positive outcomes and a life full of vitality and abundance.

In summary, the Six Factors of Intelligence give you power. They give you the ability to:

1) Choose a new response to food and to life.
2) Program your brain to actually crave healthy food.
3) Transform the image you have of yourself.
4) Know that what you imagine for yourself and your family will come true.
5) Willfully take a stand for what you want and who you want to be.
6) Step into a whole new way of being.

Without accessing these Six Intellectual Factors, you move into the next deadly myth...DENIAL.

Myth #3: Being fat isn't really that big of a deal.

If you are denying the gravity of your situation, then you are not present to the risks of being fat. There are many and they are serious.

FACT: Denial is one of the most insidious causes of obesity.

When you're caught up in the Dieting Dance and you're using

willpower to keep you committed to one diet after another, you eventually give up the dance and move into denying that you even have a weight problem, much less a serious health condition.

The natural next step in the Dieting Dance is to deny the gravity of your situation. Most people don't want to get present to the risks of being fat.

I started having stomach problems when I was nine years old. My parents didn't know because I was too ashamed to tell them. Instead, I suffered alone thinking I was bad for not having control over my bowels. Imagine what that felt like as a young girl.

Left unchecked, these symptoms turned into more serious stomach problems. I spent my late twenties getting scoped, probed, and medicated to deal with the daily pain and discomfort. As a nutritionist, I knew that my eating patterns as a child completely compromised my system in all areas.

At the age of thirty I was diagnosed with hypothyroidism, whose symptoms include depression, fatigue, and an inability to lose weight. Some days I was so exhausted, I could have slept in the middle of a busy street. The fatigue and the inability to cope made me even more stressed, which exacerbated the stomach symptoms.

This not only compromised my lifestyle, sadly it compromised my marriage. I barely had the energy to have a conversation, so sex was pretty much out of the question. I began to isolate myself from friends, and I slowly slipped into the lonely states of fear and frustration.

I didn't give up, though. Finally the thyroid medication kicked in, and my body started to regulate. Although my stomach issues persisted, I did have more energy and things were looking up.

So, my (former) husband and I decided to have a baby.

Which brought on a new problem. My years of high-sugar foods and doing the Dieting Dance also led to a condition called PCOS – Polycystic Ovary Syndrome – which results from your body's resistance to the hormone insulin. This condition can significantly impact fertility, so I had problems getting pregnant.

Once again, I felt that in some way I was inherently flawed.

For any of you who have experienced infertility, you know how deflating this can be. For some women with PCOS, it takes years to conceive. In unfortunate cases, it may never happen at all. And when your clock is ticking, there is a deep physical and emotional yearning for a child. When you don't get pregnant, month after month, it is like a big kick in the gut.

I had it easier than most. My story has a good ending.

With the help of acupuncture and a low dose of fertility medication, I got pregnant. With the shift in my hormones during pregnancy, my thyroid went into overdrive, so my doctor took me off the thyroid medication. Max was born on February 20, 2003. My stomach issues disappeared shortly thereafter, and I lost my pregnancy weight by maintaining a healthy diet and exercising daily.

Despite the overall improvements in my health, I still need to closely regulate my hormones. My history continues to put me at higher risk for things like cardiovascular disease and cancer. I am at a much lesser risk because of the healthy habits I have embraced, but it will take a lifelong effort to keep my health risks in check.

Fortunately I can take my experience and help others find their way.

As a nutritionist, I have coached hundreds of families, and the biggest hurdle we overcome is denial. Parents are so worried that talking about food will give their kids a complex about food that they avoid the subject all together.

Well, guess what? If you have a fat kid or one that is overeating or making poor food choices, then your child already has a complex around food – it's called the Fat Kid Mentality. Your taking action and talking about it actually *erases* this way of thinking.

More importantly, taking action saves lives.

When heart disease is diagnosed in someone age fifty, it didn't just show up at age fifty. It has been developing over a lifetime of poor eating and a sedentary lifestyle.

What is the starting line? It's your child's first bite of solid food.

But you want to know what's really scary? These days, eight-year-olds are diagnosed with high blood pressure, high cholesterol, and diabetes.

Do you really want to wait until you see those scary numbers on a set of lab results before you take action?

I had this conversation with one of my clients.

Her teenage son was about 100 pounds overweight, and his triglycerides and other pre-diabetic markers were off the charts. He was completely sedentary and spent most afternoons playing video games and watching TV.

While sitting in my office, after showing me the labs, she said to me, "I know this is bad. I know I need to do something, but we've tried everything, and I just don't want to make food or his weight a big deal."

I loved this woman, and I loved her son. I loved them enough to take a stand. So I gently, yet with great conviction, said, "Susan, this is already a big deal. Your son has made food and his weight a very big deal. In fact, he lives his life for the next meal, the next snack, and whether or not there is going to be enough food to go around at the dinner table. He hates going to school because he feels embarrassed walking down the halls. You may think that if you bring this to his attention he will just eat more. He's going to eat more regardless of whether you say something or not. That's because his actions aren't based on what you ARE doing; his actions are based on what you are NOT doing. He is crying out, "MOM, THIS IS A BIG DEAL! I AM FAT AND I HATE MY BODY AND I NEED HELP."

She got it. For the next twelve weeks, I went to their home and spent an hour at their kitchen table, teaching them how to lovingly make their health and their life a big deal.

So, what might happen if you make your child's weight a "big deal"?

I know it's scary. I know the Fat Kid Mentality says "you are loved only if you are skinny." I know how talking about food can spiral into negative patterns around food.

But here's the reality:

You wouldn't let your kids run out in the middle of a busy street, would you? No, you want to protect them from getting hit by a car!

What is the difference, then, in letting your kids continue habits that will hit them with the dangers of obesity? Dangers like diabetes, cancer, and Alzheimer's, or more lifelong complaints like depression, fatigue, gastrointestinal disorders, asthma, arthritis, insomnia, inflammation, infertility, migraines, adult-acne, female facial hair, PMS, and more.

Whew, it's exhausting to think about.

Now, are you ready for the next reality?

Kids are following the Fat Kid Mentality of adults.

They are too young to know this, but like you, they are eating out of self-loathing or a desire to escape.

I didn't know this as a child, but now I understand why I ate the way I did.

I recall the horrors of going to the mall to buy a bathing suit. I stood in the dressing room absolutely detesting my body. I would cry because I felt disgusting, while my mom tried to convince me that I was beautiful.

I truly love her for that, but at the time it didn't fit my belief system and all I could do was reject what she was saying. Think about it. How many times has someone said to you, "You are perfect just the way you are"?

Did it work?

Do you tell your daughter she's perfect even though she's getting teased on the playground because she's fat? Have you tried to convince your nephew he's just fine even though he's the last one chosen for the kickball team because he can't run? Do you try to convince yourself that you'll get healthy next week as you reach for your diet pills?

Denial is hard to see when you're living in it. You give it another name: "justification." You justify the situation because you don't want to deal with the discomfort of talking about the truth.

When you are in denial, you withhold the very tools that will set you – and the kids in your life – free.

Okay, let's make a change. Let's end the vicious cycle of the Dieting Dance. First, let's look at the part of the dieting definition that I embrace:

Diet = Eating in a regulated fashion.

For most, this has a negative connotation. You assume that if you are regulating what you are eating, then you are dieting.

So let's change the verbiage. How about we say you are being **mindful** of what you eat. You are **paying attention** to the choices you make. You are **aware** of what goes in your mouth. You are **watching** your portions instead of assuming seconds are just a natural part of your meal.

Meditate on those words:

- Mindful
- Paying Attention
- Aware
- Watching

Do you see the power you give yourself when you are PRESENT to the process of fueling your body (which is also called "eating")?

I regulate what I eat every day. But I'm not dieting.

I know that I need to eat breakfast to balance my hormones and stave of disease. So I give myself enough time in the morning to make a quick but healthy breakfast to share with my son.

That's being Mindful.

I allot time every week to go to the store and stock up on a week's worth of food. I make sure I have enough time so that I can read labels and ensure we're not eating too much fat, sugar, or preservatives.

That's Paying Attention.

I know I need to eat every four hours to keep my metabolism burning and to supply my brain with life-giving nutrients. So, I keep healthy snacks at my desk, in my car, and in my purse at all times.

That's being Aware.

I know if I eat big portions, I gain weight. So I eat portions that I know will promote a healthy body composition and allow myself occasional splurges to enjoy life's pleasures.

That's Watching.

Does that make sense? You can do that too! When you are Mindful, Paying Attention, Aware, and Watching how you fuel your body, you win!

Please realize I made these changes slowly over time, knowing they needed to become so much a part of ME that I would do them without thinking.

So if you really want to lose fat, attain your ideal weight, and live a healthy lifestyle, there's only one diet for you. It's the diet that honors these five truths:

1) Your body is designed to perfectly regulate itself.
2) God put wonderful foods on this planet for us to enjoy in moderation.
3) When your needs are being met through self-love and

purpose, you won't rely on the artificial high of sugar and other stimulants.

4) The body's natural inclination is to be in constant movement, so exercise is a natural desire.

5) Forcing results goes against your body's inherent ability to achieve healthy weight with ease.

Do you see how these five truths illustrate a different mindset than one focused on dieting?

We are dynamic and brilliant human beings, each with a unique body, an intricate mind, and a divine spirit. When we honor all of these and come up with ways to actualize good health habits with a **Small Change, Big Impact**™ lifestyle, then we create what everyone really wants – TRUE HEALTH and HAPPINESS.

So here's what you need to do:

Retrain your brain and radically shift your physiology.

You need to send new messages to your body so that it will return to perfect function. You need to shift your thinking away from the Fat Kid Mentality so that positive energy and thoughts become your platform. You need to pay attention and create new ways of caring for your body and walking powerfully in the world!

If you believe you can have this – true health and happiness through the **Small Change, Big Impact**™ lifestyle that I'm going to prescribe – then you are ready to take the next step.

I invite you to take on these fourteen Daily Lessons to break through your Fat Kid Mentality. I guarantee that, through the messages on these pages, you will completely transform your life.

Daily Lesson #1:
CHANGE YOUR FEATURE ATTRACTIONS (SELF-VIEW)

Before we get started on our journey together, I want you to stop for a moment...take a deep breath...and answer this question:

What is my desired outcome in mastering these Fourteen Daily Lessons to Break Through the Fat Kid Mentality?

Come up with your own answer and write it here:

_____

_____

If you wrote, "Because I want to lose weight," then take a moment to think about **why** you want to lose weight.

For many of you, losing weight will make you feel better about yourself. You've decided that by being a certain weight, you fit a set of standards that allows you to be kinder and more accepting of yourself.

Or you may feel that by losing weight you can get **others** to feel better about you. Possibly your husband, girlfriend, boss, or friend show more love and respect if you lose weight.

These reasons are quite common. I also know, through years of experience, that these reasons are deadly. Wanting to lose weight as a way to earn love and respect furthers the Fat Kid Mentality that says, "You will only be accepted if you meet a certain set of standards."

With this mentality, you can't win.

Rather, your motivation should be based on reclaiming that which is rightfully yours – perfect health, energy, vitality, and all the things that keep you in a state of self-love. In other words, this new motivation is the difference between thinking **"I'm not good enough so I must change"** to **"BECAUSE I'm good enough, I must change."**

You simply cannot have other people as your motivation for losing weight or getting fit. The desire must come from you and be accomplished for you.

Here's the shift. If you can embrace this very first Daily Lesson, then the next thirteen lessons will truly set you free. They will give you the power to unequivocally govern your health for the rest of your life.

But it starts with this first critical step:

Change your view of yourself.

Wow, sounds like a big job, right? You've been walking around for years with the same self-view and now I'm asking you to poof – change it!

I know this is not easy. If it were, then everyone would be do-ing it and we wouldn't be having this conversation. But here's the deal. You are ready for this! You are the one who is going to do it differently and stop the madness. I know this because there are no accidents, and you are the one holding this book.

Now, I have one request of you.

If you are launching into this book feeling unmotivated, un-educated, unhappy, unworthy, UN-anything...then this will just be another one of those books on your shelf.

If you decide, however, to step into new beliefs about yourself – to break through the Fat Kid Mentality and build a new view about yourself – then this book will change your life. Next year this book will be so tattered and torn that you'll need to duct-tape the heck out of it just to keep it from falling apart. THAT'S how much this philosophy will become a part of your life.

Remind yourself why you are here.

For instance, do you like walking into a store and feeling like everyone is staring at you because you're overweight? NO. And by the way, they aren't staring – you just think they are because this is how you see yourself.

What if you saw yourself as beautiful, sexy, confident, and pow-erful? Now you walk into a store and feel people staring at you because you are so amazing! And by the way, they aren't staring at you – you just think they are because this is how you see yourself.

So either way, you are going to feel like people are checking you out in judgment – good or bad. Whether it's how you look, talk, drive your car, or run a meeting...people's eyes are upon you.

Now, this is all fantasy. People are not checking you out. YOU are checking you out. If you are checking yourself out as someone who is motivated, committed, sensible, and capable of making permanent change, then this is how the world sees you too.

And, this is how you will take on the Daily Lessons in this book.

The coolest part is that YOU get to decide! You get to choose which traits or attractions you want to feature to the world every day. Let's say you're writing a screenplay that everyone is going to watch. In marketing yourself to the world, what wonderful parts are you going to share to sell the tickets?

You could say, "This is boring, unmotivating, and will pretty much leave you feeling empty and bitter." Hmmm, not too enticing. So scrap those statements and start over.

Try this on: "This is exhilarating, funny, bright, inspiring, and will make you feel like you could jump right in and be instant friends with the main character!" Yes, you'd want to check that out!

The other day my mom gave me a beautiful book. It is a collection of stories and quotes that my grandmother collected over the years. I found this excerpt and feel it fits here perfectly:

"A woman's figure? Of course I notice it. But I see it through the impressions already formed – impressions which can alter, magically, a good figure into a perfect one."

You form the impressions you have of yourself, and that's what the world reflects back to you. It's time to form new impressions. It's time to LET GO of every negative self-trait you believe and define the FEATURE ATTRACTIONS that will set a new stage.

Here's how you do it.

SMALL CHANGE:

It's list-making time. Get out a blank piece of paper and set aside some quiet time – about twenty minutes or more. You can put on your favorite music, light a candle, or find a shady spot under a tree. Create a positive environment for yourself and be willing to close your eyes for a moment.

First, imagine you are leaving your body and taking a seat across from yourself. If this feels too strange, imagine you are already standing a few feet away. In this scenario, you are your best friend, just hanging out and helping make this list.

The reason I'm having you be your friend, rather than picturing someone else, is that you have wonderful traits that you have kept secret – although not intentionally – even from your closest friends. Yet in focusing on the negative traits, you have unknowingly kept the lovely ones hidden. So try not to stand in other people's shoes but in your own shoes, looking in.

Now start making a list of all your FEATURE ATTRACTIONS – those brilliant and wonderful traits that you were born with and could light up a room if given the chance. In helping to make this list, what would your friend say? Here are some suggestions to help get you started:

I am as loyal to myself as I am to others.

I have a perfect body that is just waiting to be uncovered and shown to the world.

I have an unwavering faith in myself to get the job done.

I am generous with myself.

I am brave.

Come up with as many statements at possible. There are no set rules or requirements, but I would encourage you to think of at least ten. If you need to set down the list and pick it up at a later time, that's fine too. But if you're on a roll, just go for it! No one is watching – just you, and well, you.

Be honest. Be authentic. Be bold. Don't hold back. This is your time. THIS is your first step to moving beyond the Dieting Dance forever! This is how you change your view of yourself. This is how you save your life and the lives of those around you.

BIG IMPACT:

I know what it's like to withhold Feature Attractions and walk around with a negative self-view. I did it too.

For most of my teenage years, I walked to school every day feeling like everyone was checking me out. I heard "She's gained weight," "Look at that double-chin," "Her clothes are too tight," "Look at her skinny friend next to her." Yuck.

I know you can imagine what this feels like. It's torture – especially when you know, on some deeper level, that people don't really know who you are. Sure, I was always the funny one. I still hung out with the popular crowd, and people thought I had a great smile and got along with everyone. I was nice.

But people were really missing out! For the longest time I never shared, in depth, my capacity for love. I have SO much love to give, but I never let on to this, even with my parents and my dearest friends.

When I was about twenty-five, I started doing some personal work that helped me view my life in a different way. One day I sat down and made my list of Feature Attractions. I "looked in" at myself, as I'm asking you to do in this exercise, and thought, "Wow, you really know how to love people."

Then I thought, "Well, everyone knows this, so I don't need to write this down." But when I really thought about it, I wondered if people *did* know how much I could love them.

I started making a list of how I show my love to the people who are closest to me. I came up with about five ways and realized the list was painfully short compared to all the ways I **knew** I could love. As I thought about this, I came up with a very short statement:

"I am love."

That was it. I – AM – LOVE. This statement became my number one Feature Attraction and grew more profound for me over the years. I created an exponential shift in my thinking. Do you think in stating "I Am Love" I could also say, "Well, I am love, but I hate myself and my body"? Um, no. That's not possible.

If I am love, then there is no room for hate. And if there's no room for hate, then there's no room for hating my body. So, with this statement as my coach, I began to hate my body less and love people more.

However, I would be lying if I said that all of a sudden I LOVED my body and never had a negative self-view again.

Still, the statement "I am love" does provide a reference point every time I have this self-defeating thought. "I am love" moves me out of anything that has to do with hate. With practice, this has become the very measure for choices I make around food, exercise, meditation, stress, and my relationship to others.

Let's say you start reading the following pages with the belief "I hate my body, and if I can just lose the weight, then I'll like myself again and others will like me too."

How successful do you think you would be in allowing this book to change your self-view?

If this is how you currently operate, then any time you feel frustrated, tired, angry, hungry, deprived, or whatever comes up for you, you will close the book and walk away forever.

Instead, every time you experience one of these feelings, you can refer to your Feature Attractions list and apply your statements: "I am love," "I am brave," "I am loyal to myself," "I am committed to taking a stand for my children."

Do you see how this sets you up for success?

Different view, different results.

Once you have made your list, you will have it for a lifetime. It becomes every bit a part of how you walk in the world as a complete and whole person. Even if all you do is write down one Feature Attraction and say this over and over to yourself daily, you are breaking through the Fat Kid Mentality that says "You are not worth seeing."

Now, take your Feature Attraction list and use it as your bookmark as you read through the remainder of the lessons and let's get on with Daily Lesson #2 where we'll be talking about how you can befriend food.

Daily Lesson #2:
BEFRIEND FOOD

What does it mean to befriend food?

You already *love* food, right? In fact, you love food so much you believe it's the reason you're overweight. How do I know this? Because you are not unlike many of my overweight clients who say to me, "If I just didn't love food so much, I'd be skinny."

But do you *really* love food?

What about when you feel unhappy about your weight? How do you feel about food then? Is food your friend when being fat makes you feel depressed, anxious, unloved, and unaccepted?

Wouldn't you agree that when you are unhappy, food then becomes the enemy?

If you answered yes, consider this.

This enemy (food) is so pervasive that every time you order a meal, put an item in your grocery cart, or eat from the holiday buffet, your Fat Kid Mentality says,

"I am eating food, so I am bad."

And what's even more deadening is that once food becomes the enemy, it doesn't matter whether it's a carrot, a brownie, an apple, or a potato.

The idea that you are eating at all makes you bad!

This is all part of your Fat Kid Mentality.

This mentality is the belief that food is bad or at least something to be reckoned with.

But food is not bad. Food is vital. And wonderfully prepared foods that are eaten in proper portions can be one of life's greatest pleasures.

Just the other morning I enjoyed a beautiful meal my boyfriend made for me. It was a gorgeous display of homemade crepes stuffed with sautéed apples, pears, and bananas sprinkled with cinnamon.

I had two small crepes and some green tea with honey. It was glorious!

If I were still stuck in my Fat Kid Mentality, I could have easily slipped into the trap of "food as the enemy" *and suffered through every bite.* That would have taken me completely out of the moment and kept me from appreciating all the love that went into preparing this nutritious meal with splendidly fresh food.

Can you relate?

The first step in befriending food is to realize that food is not the enemy, but that your **thoughts** around food are the enemy. When you identify your thoughts, you will see the negative connotations around food that include:

1) confusion
2) seduction
3) addiction
4) guilt
5) punishment
6) shame
7) fear
8) failure
9) illness
10) pain

When you have these beliefs around food, there is no way you can enjoy your meals. You will judge everything you put in your mouth, every moment of every day.

And you are not alone.

In fact, EVERYONE – the fat, the fit, and the in-between – has some sort of limiting idea around food. This is why I say that every-one has a Fat Kid Mentality.

As an experiment, start observing how this mentality plays out with your friends.

Your fat friends will admit to being bad when they eat potato chips, order the burger, or go for round two at the BBQ. They boldly state they have no control over the "enemy" and resign themselves to the idea that food is making them fat and unhappy.

On the other hand, your skinny friends will proudly say they *ward off* the enemy. They'll proclaim that dessert is bad, nuts are addicting, and bread is dangerous.

Yet interestingly, in the same breath, they'll admit to **loving** dessert, **revering** nuts, and **craving** bread. The difference is that they **don't eat any of these** because they don't want to feel guilty and bad. So guess what happens when they occasionally acquiesce and eat these foods. They deal with the Fat Kid Mentality that says, "The enemy just got the best of you."

Somewhere in your youth you bought into the societal messages around being fat. So you were either defeated by the message and went on to become a fat adult or you were the skinny one who vowed to battle the enemy and overcome it with your martyred avoidance.

I don't know about you, but neither one of these beliefs sounds particularly fun to me.

That's why I'm teaching you how to befriend food, so you can dispose of these defeating thoughts and start enjoying the foods that were so graciously placed on this planet.

And you will see that when you befriend food, it's not just something you do. Rather, it becomes a lifestyle.

To this day, despite my healthy mindset, I need to consciously befriend food every time I get ice cream with my son Max. If I didn't do this, and instead felt guilty eating ice cream, then I would be buying into the idea that food is the enemy. This mentality would destroy the enjoyment I get out of this fun outing with my son.

I also befriend food every time I eat a piece of bread. I befriend food when I eat a late-night bowl of cereal. I befriend food when I eat a piece of cake.

In the past, eating these foods would have made me bad. Now I make the decision to embrace them, savor them, appreciate them, and honor them as foods that I consciously choose.

And you know why I'm okay with this?

Because this is what I needed to do when I decided to transform *my* Fat Kid Mentality and embrace the pleasures and joys around some of my favorite foods.

You will see in the Big Impact story below that this did not happen in college when I started running eight blocks. It did not happen when I went back to school to study nutrition. It happened much later.

So I'm inviting you to let go of any notions you have about your place in this process. Let it all go! Today, whether you're fat or thin, you will break through the belief that food is bad and rid yourself of this mentality forever.

SMALL CHANGE:

So to begin befriending your food, you must first define what you want food to represent for you. In doing so, you will naturally choose foods that support a friendly outcome.

Before I lead you into the exercise, you must agree to this important premise and **make it your mantra:**

Food is on the planet for my pleasure and my health.

Say that again:

Food is on the planet for my pleasure and my health.

Say this over and over until it becomes your own. It may seem difficult at first to truly believe this, but if you can make it your own truth, you will have new possibilities around eating that will result in healthy weight.

Now for the next step.

Take out a piece of paper and fold it in half vertically to make two columns. On the left-hand column, make a list of the foods that are most prominent in your diet. This can be anything. If an apple is in your diet, write it down. If ice cream is in your diet, write it down. Beef, sunflower seeds, wine, milk...whatever you eat or drink, write it down.

Now that you've made your list, in the right-hand column next to each food or beverage item, I want you to write down what each one represents to you as it relates to your mantra above:

Health or Pleasure.

You can have more than one association with a particular food. For example, for me, apples represent Health and Pleasure, whereas ice cream represents only Pleasure. So next to apples I'd write Health/Pleasure and next to ice cream I'd write Pleasure.

There are no right or wrong answers. This is for YOU to decide your reasons for choosing the foods that you do. What we'll achieve is a shift in your mindset from "food is the enemy" to **"food is here on the planet for my pleasure and my health."**

When you believe this, it's a win-win!

And better yet, you will move into a place where you make empowered choices. you are choosing this: "Do I want to eat this for Health, Pleasure, or both?"

Just in doing this exercise, you will shift your relationship to food. You will take responsibility for choosing some foods for pleasure but not necessarily for health. Does this make food bad? No! It's just YOUR CHOICE in that moment, which will in turn make you more mindful of your choices.

I am not asking you to go down your list and write whether each food is good or bad. I'm just asking you to be *real* about your choices and decide how much of the pleasure/health combinations you want in your life.

The fact is, when you have both pleasure and health in more of your choices, you will feel better and be more balanced.

For example, if I ate only healthy foods like apples all the time, I would miss out on pleasurable experiences like eating ice cream. On the flip side, if I chose ice cream all the time, I would miss out on the vibrant health I enjoy from foods like apples that allow me to maintain my weight and live an amazing life.

What this exercise does is remove all the negative connotations around food so that you are empowered to make choices based on two simple premises:

Pleasure and Health.

In creating a balance between the two, you move away from the negative associations around food and embrace new ones where food represents:

1) health
2) vitality
3) fun
4) family
5) tradition

6) joy
7) creativity
8) commitment
9) abundance
10) pleasure

Those are friendlier terms, don't you think?

Here's what happened when I did this exercise and chose to befriend food.

BIG IMPACT:

I had just started my nutrition practice.

I knew I had a powerful message to share and that my teachings were going to change people's lives. I was "walking my talk," living a clean and healthy life, and it showed. I was 5'4' and 118 pounds – a far cry from the fat girl who started running eight blocks in college.

Well, unbeknownst to me, that fat girl was still hangin' out. But I didn't realize this until I started listening to the stories of my clients. Day after day I'd listen to proclamations of self-hate, despair, and the entrapment of battles with food.

For the first three months in practice I came home every night and cried. Despite my colleagues' warnings to not get attached to my clients, I was taking every one of their stories to heart. There were days when the accounts of their lives were so overwhelming that I felt completely defeated. I would think to myself, "There is no way I can heal this depth of pain."

Then one day, my spiritual teacher asked me, "Julie, why do you think you are feeling so sad about your clients' stories?"

I thought about it for a few moments. I looked up and said, "Because their stories are mine."

It was in that moment that I realized I was still living in a world of despair around my relationship to food. Even though I was a healthy weight, I was still entrenched in the mentality that food was the enemy.

To be clear, I wasn't dieting during this time. I wasn't restricting calories or following some fad plan. Rather, I was committed to teaching my clients about foundation nutrition and how to choose healthy foods with ease.

The missing piece was that I was not being honest about the guilt that still came up every time I had a few bites of cake or had seconds on pasta or even put too much fruit in my smoothies, for goodness sake!

So when I heard these same stories from my clients, it really hit home that I needed to change my own ways before I could empower others to change theirs. I didn't want health to be a constant struggle, and I didn't want that for my clients either.

So I had to heal myself. And in doing so, I had to let go of my old paradigms around food – to start enjoying food instead of judging it.

For many months I thought about how I could make the shift. I worked with my teacher, read books, went to seminars, listened to CDs....wow, it was just too much work.

Then one day I was sitting in silence, a practice I've committed to daily. During this time, I asked the question, "What does food represent to me?" I came up with the negative qualities as previously listed above:

1) confusion
2) seduction
3) addiction
4) guilt
5) punishment
6) shame
7) fear
8) failure
9) illness
10) pain

I started to sob. Wow, did I really think all these things every time I thought about food?

Yes.

So then I asked myself, "What do I *want* food to represent for me?" And I came up with the positive definitions as previously listed above:

1) celebration
2) vitality
3) fun
4) family
5) tradition
6) joy
7) creativity
8) commitment
9) abundance
10) flavor

This made me feel lighter and instilled hope.

Then I thought, "Okay, how do I get to the place where food

will naturally represent the friendlier outcomes?" I sat in silence. Then the word "health" came to me. And I smiled and thought, "Yes, food represents health." But this didn't seem to be the complete answer. So I stayed open to more insight. Then a new word came to me..."pleasure." I was stunned. Wow, is it possible that food could be here as both health *and* pleasure?

Then I thought about the foods that are supposedly bad but give me pleasure. It was then that I realized my Fat Kid Mentality was talking. It was basically instilling the belief that certain foods needed to be labeled as bad, even if they were pleasurable.

But if it's MY choice, can't I decide to define food differently? Isn't it in my power to choose food for health or pleasure?

So I made my list.

I wrote out all the foods that show up in my diet in the left-hand column, which include things like bananas, eggs, kale, and yams but also cinnamon ice cream, potato salad, chocolate, wedding cake, and freshly baked bread.

I then went down the right side of the column and wrote the words "health" or "pleasure" next to each food, as I've instructed you to do above. It was remarkable!

I saw bananas as health and pleasure.

Ice cream as pleasure.

Kale as health.

Chocolate as health and pleasure.

I kept going down my list.

Wedding cake...sheer pleasure.

I got to the bottom of my list and realized that nowhere on my paper was the word "bad." Everything on my list was either for health, pleasure, or both. The negative judgments towards certain foods had completely lifted.

I felt really good about that. I also felt okay that there were certain foods I ate simply because they were good for me – such as kale. I'm not so psyched about kale, but I MAKE THE CHOICE to eat it because I know it's good for me, not because someone is forcing me to do it. And then with the ice cream and wedding cake... "Go for it, Julie, they give you pleasure!"

This was one of the most freeing moments in my life.

I looked at that list over and over and felt such joy and release in knowing that food did not need to be the enemy.

The next time I ate a piece of bread, I just savored and celebrated every last morsel. I could join the rest of the people at the table in saying, "Wow, isn't this bread amazing?"

The next time I ordered ice cream I thought, "I am so fortunate that I can have this wonderful treat and still enjoy good health." I would talk about the flavors and the sweetness and the creaminess...and not once did I think, "This is so bad, but I'm doing it anyway."

What freedom!

Now, as said before, I still consciously befriend food every now and then. When I hear those old thought patterns coming up, I remind myself of the mantra:

Food is on this planet for my pleasure and my health.

Do you see how easy this can be? It's about choice. It's about
a lifestyle. It's about your WORDS. It's about deciding that your
world around food can be GOOD and supportive and nurturing in
all aspects of life...mind, body, and spirit.

Believe me, when you do this, you will never abuse that privilege. You will choose health and pleasure in moderation, break
through the Fat Kid Mentality, and listen to the wisdom of your
body that says:

Food is your friend.

ENROLL OTHERS AND BUILD T.E.A.M.

S o often people who want to lose weight convince themselves that to be successful, they must forge ahead on their own.

Does this sound familiar?

Do you believe that creating a new healthy life is your sole responsibility, and that others are not to be bothered by your concerns?

If you live life this way, know that it's a trap, especially with your health. If you want to break free from the Fat Kid Mentality, you need to ask for help.

Cutting people out of your process to lose weight has nothing to do with protecting them from your problems. It has nothing to do with keeping you safe from criticism, or even about being valiant. It's not even about being subdued or keeping yourself out of the limelight.

This is about something much deeper.

Because when you don't ask for help, you are keeping yourself stuck in the Fat Kid Mentality that says, "Nobody cares."

I want you to really think about this. Listen to how devaluing that statement is:

"Nobody cares."

First, it implies that nobody cares about *you*.

Second, saying that "nobody cares" suggests that people are generally uncaring.

If you agree with what I'm saying, then ask yourself these two questions:

1) Do you *believe* that nobody cares about you?

2) Do you *believe* that people don't care in general?

I know at times it may feel true that nobody cares. And in fact, there are people in your life who are more concerned with themselves than they are about you.

But for the most part, the reason you feel people don't care is because you haven't given them the *opportunity* to care.

That's right. People don't seem to care, because you have not successfully enrolled them in the importance of your mission to get healthy. You have not opened your heart to them, to share your vulnerabilities or your limitations. You have not given them credit for being someone who can move you toward higher levels of success. You have not allowed people to PLAY BIG and share of themselves in ways that bring out the best in you.

Does any of this ring true for you? Do you see how the Fat Kid Mentality of "nobody cares" sabotages your efforts by shutting people out? And do you see that in doing so, you not only lose your own power, but you take away power from the people who care about you the most?

Don't worry. You are not alone. I continue to work on this part of my Fat Kid Mentality every day.

It has been a big lesson for me to see how I thwart my efforts toward greatness by trying to figure out things on my own. I work over problems in my head – ruminating for hours – and then never share a single ounce of what I'm feeling with those around me.

When I'm in the midst of a problem, I will think to myself, "I don't want anyone to know that I am weak" or "I don't want people to think I'm irresponsible" or "I need to be an inspiration to others."

Wow, what a heavy load to bear.

Yet when I choose to share my feelings of confusion or fear, the people in my life reach out to me in incredible ways – with love, compassion, and unwavering respect. They don't see me as weak but feel honored to be part of what I'm powerfully creating. They don't see me as irresponsible but recognize that my "humanness" makes me more approachable. They don't see me as less of an inspiration but more as a catalyst for their own change and personal growth.

It's quite remarkable. People want to help you. Yet often they won't do it unless you give them permission. You need to ask. You need to let them in.

So what about you? Are you afraid to ask for help? And does this fear keep you resigned to staying the way you are?

Let today be your day to seek help, enroll others, and build a team of people who are on your side to win.

I'm going to teach you how to build your T.E.A.M. I use this acronym because there are four critical steps to getting people involved in your process, as spelled out below. The acronym will help you remember the steps so that they become habit.

SMALL CHANGE:

T = Trust

The trust starts the minute you tell someone you are committed to changing your life.

This is a big step to take, but you can do it. Don't ever look back or over-think this step. Just go with your instincts of who you'd like to support you through this process.

The best way to do this is to take the next twenty seconds to write down five names. Go with your gut. Write down the first five names that come to mind, without judgment or thoughts of past experiences. You just know, in this moment, that if it came to life or death, you could trust these five people.

Set your timer for twenty seconds. Get prepared to write. Take a deep breath. Ready...Set...GO!

1.
2.
3.

4.

5.

Look at your list again and get present to the people you've chosen. Don't erase or add anybody yet. Don't over-analyze your choices. Just know that you inherently trust these people and have now chosen them for your T.E.A.M.

You can do this exercise again and choose others. In fact you may seek out new team members that may include a doctor, a personal trainer, a spiritual counselor, or even a new friend. I encourage you, however, not to exclude anyone from your lists.

What you have done now is create an environment of openness. You have solidified an unwavering faith, knowing that what you share with these people will bring forth the results you desire.

E = Empathy

As a nutritionist, I practice empathy in my job every day. I call it "mirroring." When someone is struggling, rather than talking her out of the pain, I mirror back her distress or worries.

I will use phrases like:

"I see that you are really struggling, and I know this can be difficult."

Or

"I am sorry you are feeling frustrated right now."

These empathic responses are much more empowering than:

"You worry too much."

Or,

"You're not trying hard enough."

When people discount your feelings with judgment, they are not meeting you at the place where you can work together on a solution. They are giving you the answer by saying, "Get over it."

Remember this when you're asking others for help. You can use this mirroring, or this empathy, to invite others into your life in a way that suits them. Rather than pointing out where they have done you wrong, or assuming they are going to be inconvenienced, start by having empathy for them and admitting how you have shut them out.

For example:

"I know I've been blaming you for my weight, and I want you to know I notice that. I'm doing something different now, and I'd really love your help."

OR

"I know you get frustrated when I'm in a bad mood around my weight. And I realize that must be really hard for you. I'd love to share some of the things I'm doing differently now. I'm really excited about it, and I know I'll be more successful if you're here to help me."

OR

"I know I have been skeptical of your advice and I realize that may cause you to shut down. I am ready to make some significant changes in my life and I have chosen you for my team. I would be honored if you would continue to offer your support."

With these statements, you are showing empathy for the other person by mirroring their feelings. You are also showing empathy for yourself by having an authentic and meaningful conversation. What a loving gesture toward them and also for yourself.

You will be pleasantly surprised when people put their agendas aside and offer genuine support. This gives you a chance to be okay with what you are feeling. And when your feelings are supported, you will spend less time evaluating what's wrong and more time coming up with solutions.

A = Attitude Adjustment

Think of a piano. When one key is off, the melody changes. This doesn't mean you get rid of the key. That one key is an important part of the instrument. Rather, you simply tune the key, and the slight adjustment creates a beautiful song.

You are no different.

You are going to have days when you feel off key. You'll have moments when you feel out of harmony with what you are trying to accomplish. You'll feel negative, discouraged, tired, and frustrated.

That's okay and is to be expected.

The problem starts when those feelings spread or stick around for too long. That's when you call on your T.E.A.M. for the fine-tuning. Call for motivation. Call for inspiration. Call for help in making the slight shifts in your attitude so that you can see your world a little differently.

This is why you have your T.E.A.M.! Allow them to offer what they do best. Some of your team members will just offer a hug or a word of insight. Others might get you out for a walk or suggest a helpful book. Others may practice more tough love and get you out of your funk with a loving kick in the pants.

Whatever it may be, embrace it. Don't take the slight shifts in attitude for granted. Sometimes it may take only twenty minutes to get you back in tune and aligned with the actions steps that get you moving forward.

M = Manage Up

I'm always open to the wisdom and teachings of my clients.

In fact, sometimes our best work happens when they show me something I either overlooked or discounted because I thought I knew it all.

This is not a hierarchical system. You and your T.E.A.M. will benefit greatly from humbly voicing your concerns and giving your honest feedback.

So, when your spouse fails to get home on time for you to get to the gym, you can say, "It seems like the schedule we laid out is not working. I am committed to getting to the gym, and you are committed to getting home on time so that I can do that. Do we need to look at a different plan? I'd be happy to explore this, but I would prefer if you could re-commit to the plan we have in place."

In this scenario, you have stated your commitment to get to the gym, and that you expect your partner to follow through with his commitment as well. You have not let pride or ridicule turn your request into a demand but have simply suggested that you both come up with a way to stay mutually committed.

I realize these types of conversations can be scary. I know that you don't want to get people upset or angry. So the trick is to stay calm, use a loving but firm tone, and remain true to yourself and your commitment.

Allow yourself to ask for help, but also be an inspiration.

By keeping others committed, you are giving them the gift of knowing you. They know you by knowing what you want. When they see that YOU are consistent and that you are enrolling other committed people, they will not want to miss out on being part of your T.E.A.M.

BIG IMPACT

My client George is a strong-willed, independent, and successful owner of a multimillion dollar company.

He is married, with three children, and is very active in his community. He coaches his daughter's soccer team, volunteers at his church, and has an active social life with other successful men and women. He is a leader who in the past did not ask for help.

Yet six months after working with me and learning how to enroll others and build his T.E.A.M., George saw profound shifts in his life that resulted in a permanent weight loss of over thirty-five pounds.

When George came to see me, he had been struggling with his weight for twenty-five years. Since graduating from college, he had been gaining one to two pounds per year, and was looking at a clinical diagnosis of obesity.

He described himself as a "self-starter who can figure things out on his own." He has lost weight before but needed a diet that would fit his busy schedule. He said his wife was too busy to cook, and after work he was consumed with his kids and their school and sports. Work was incredibly demanding, so he didn't have time to exercise or eat a healthy lunch. To top it off, he had taken on a new project at his church and felt certain he was in way over his head.

After George finished this lengthy summation, we both took a deep breath and smiled.

I said, "Whew. You definitely have a lot on your plate. It seems like you might need a little help to get it all done."

He replied, "No, I really don't need help. I always get things done."

And I said, "Except for losing weight. You haven't gotten that done."

"Right," he said humbly with a smile, "I have not done that."

I asked, "Will you agree, then, to listen to one very important suggestion for how you can get that done?"

"Sure!" he responded.

"You need to let people know that you want their help," I said.

He smiled and said, "Okaaaay. What do you mean exactly?"

I explained to George that in doing everything on his own, he has not allowed people into his world. His strength and valor gave the impression that no one was capable of meeting his needs.

I asked if he'd ever told his wife how important it was that he get to a healthy weight. He said he'd complained to her about his weight but did not expect her to come up with the answers.

I shared with George that asking others for help doesn't mean they need to do the work for him or come up with the all the solutions. Rather, in sharing his challenges and his commitment with his wife, he could get her enrolled on a more supportive level. So far, all she had heard was complaining.

I also asked George if he'd ever talked to his friends or his pastor about his troubles with weight. He said he'd always been a role model to his friends and never thought about asking them for advice. He also didn't want to look "lame" in front of his pastor, although could see how his spiritual path could lead him to a new understanding around his weight.

My next question to George was how he felt about asking me for help.

He responded that he wasn't sure, but the question alone made him feel uncomfortable.

So that's where we began.

George could see in our conversation that he was reluctant to ask for help. He didn't yet understand why this was important to losing weight, but he could tell we were on to something. George signed up for my six-month coaching program, and I started bringing him through the Daily Lessons as described in this book.

For George, the first step was to build his T.E.A.M. When he started doing this, he was amazed at how many people stepped up to the plate.

His wife gave up her Wednesday night knitting class and her Thursday Pilates class so she could start making more meals at home. His assistant at work started bringing him healthy lunches to eat at his desk and enforced a no candy rule in the office so George wasn't tempted by the sugary snack bowl. His assistant coach on the soccer team suggested he start doing the drills with the girls so he could get in some added exercise. And his pastor relieved him from the church project, noting that he'd be a powerful servant to his church by showing others how to achieve optimal health.

In six months George lost thirty-eight pounds.

He was happy with his weight but admitted the real success came from softening his demeanor. By doing so, he created new relationships with the important people in his life.

He and his wife were more of a team, and it made him feel good that she could be a bigger part of his day-to-day activities. He was also leading by example at work and hired me to coach the top executives in his company. He also created open relationships with his male friends, who became a huge source of inspiration with their own efforts to get healthy.

In the past, George would have kept his weight loss regimen a secret, not wanting to burden others with what he saw as a weakness. Now he was offering a gift to others by enrolling them in his life and granting them the opportunity to play big.

When you ask for help, everybody wins. You win by accomplishing your goals, and everyone around you wins because they get the gift of you. Remember, people want to help. They want to be a part of your life.

Let them in. Enroll others and build your T.E.A.M. Start by sharing with others that you are reading this book. They will want to know more, and you will create a momentum that will bring forth amazing changes in your life and the lives of those around you.

Daily Lesson #4:
ALWAYS EAT BREAKFAST

I know you've heard this a thousand times. I also know you're not doing it.

And the reason you're not eating breakfast is because you don't understand how critical this health habit is to your life – and to your *performance throughout life.*

Whether I'm coaching people on weight loss or managing a life-threatening disease, I insist my clients commit to this practice before we do anything else.

That's how vital breakfast is to your overall health.

Your breakfast habits affect every hormonal and physiological pathway in your body. These habits set everything in motion – good or bad.

I realize the words "hormones" and "physiological" may turn you away from this conversation. You might feel these words don't apply to you or they are too clinical. But I'm giving you credit for your intelligence and also stating the facts:

Hormones and physiology DO apply to you. Yes, even if you're a man – you have hormones too.

With that said, I will give you an easier way to look at it.

When I am teaching young children, I ask them to think of their body as a car. I tell them, "If you don't put fuel in your car, it won't go."

Simple right?

Your body is no different. Without the needed fuel, your body won't operate. More importantly, **when you don't eat breakfast,** your body goes into the following destructive chain of events:

1. It breaks down muscle to release stored energy, resulting in decreased muscle mass.
2. When you lose muscle mass, your metabolism slows down to such a pace that you actually GAIN weight, despite your perception of taking in fewer calories.
3. You increase stress hormones like cortisol and adrenaline, which encourage your body to store fat.
4. You lower blood glucose levels to the point where you crave stimulants like sugar, alcohol, and caffeine.
5. Your cells become less responsive to the hormone insulin, which leads to diabetes.

Wow, did you know this? Are you feeling any different about skipping breakfast now that you know the implications?

Here's some more information that will further inform and give you ownership of what's going on in your body.

First, when you go to sleep at night, you go into fasting mode.

For six to eight hours, you give your body permission to spend less time digesting and breaking down food and more time to restore and repair. The nutrition you have received during the day does its magic as you rebuild tissue, cleanse the liver, and restore cellular health.

During this time, your blood glucose levels drop. Insulin has effectively shuttled energy from your evening meal into your muscles where it is stored in the form of glycogen. While you are sleeping, you are expending very little energy. As a result, you don't use this stored glycogen – or energy – as readily as you do during your active hours.

When you wake in the morning, your glucose levels are still low. Granted, you have this stored energy in your muscles, but your brain needs energy very quickly. As soon as you open your eyes, the brain is saying, "Give me food so I can tell the body to walk, talk, think, and move."

Quite simply, for you to function, the brain needs to function.

Sound complicated? Here's the simple answer:

Eat breakfast.

When you BREAK the FAST, automatically your body will be prompted to:

1) Supply your brain and muscles with immediate energy to perform critical tasks that dictate your entire day.
2) Maintain lean muscle mass since your brain won't need to steal energy from your muscles to function.
3) Start burning fat rather than storing it because you will have stable blood sugar and normal responses to stress.

And just like your car, you'll be giving your body the fuel it needs to operate effectively.

SMALL CHANGE:

Here are some quick and light breakfast ideas for those who need to inch toward this healthy habit. **Remember, you need to eat within thirty minutes of waking to avoid the destructive chain of events.** If that's difficult for you because you're not hungry, then at least try to eat within a one-hour window. I know this may seem difficult, but just start with something small, and over time your body will adjust.

- 2 sticks of low-fat string cheese and 1 apple or a fist-sized piece of fruit
- 1 cup unsweetened oatmeal with ½ cup milk (almond, soy or organic cow's milk), 1 T. walnuts, 1 t. honey or real maple syrup, and ½ cup of sliced fruit or berries. If you're in a real rush, make it at home and take it to work to eat at your desk.
- 1 piece whole grain toast or English muffin with 1 T. peanut or almond butter
- 1 whole-grain breakfast bar (2-4 grams of fiber per serving) with one hard-boiled egg or stick of string cheese
- 6 oz. Greek yogurt – packed with protein and low in sugar and fat – plus 1 cup berries or sliced fruit
- ½ cup low-fat cottage cheese and 1 fresh peach or 2 nectarines
- Egg-white omelet with veggies from previous night's dinner JuicePlus+® Complete vanilla shake mix, blended with 1 cup berries and one handful of baby spinach. (www.maxjuiceplus.com)
- 1 cup of lentil or black bean soup (for palates that prefer spicier foods)

- ½ cup hummus with pre-cut veggies or whole-grain crackers
- Scrambled tofu with brown rice and sauteed spinach
- 1 handful of almonds and a tangerine or fruit of choice
- Leftovers from dinner
- Organic sliced turkey sandwich on whole grain bread and sliced avocado
- Hot quinoa (keen-wa) mixed with honey, almonds, and a dash of cinnamon. You can make this more savory by adding white or black beans and salsa – make the night before if you are rushed in the morning.

For more recipes and breakfast ideas, please visit my website at www.juliehammerstein.com.

BIG IMPACT:

Kathy is a forty-one-year-old mom who wants to lose weight. She is also concerned that her daughter is emulating her "bad" habits – namely, her addiction to sugar and erratic snacking as a source of comfort. Kathy also complains of low energy, which keeps her from exercising.

She describes her days as stressful – caring for her family, managing the household, and running a part-time business from home. She admittedly meets others' needs before her own and struggles with consistently practicing self-care in the areas of exercise, diet, and rest.

Her mornings start by getting her kids off to school – packing lunch, cleaning up, carpooling to different locations for each child – and then rushing home to cram in a few hours of work before heading off to shuttle the kids to extracurricular activities.

Her biggest challenges start at 4pm, when she is so hungry

and grouchy that she resorts to grazing on cookies and chips until dinner. By the time she finally gets the kids to bed, she relaxes into two frozen fudge bars as a way to decompress and reward herself for a hard day's work.

Sound familiar?

As she sat in my office I asked, "Do you eat breakfast?" She laughed, "I don't have time to eat breakfast and to be quite honest, I don't even think about food until 11am when I'm starving and I could eat the entire pantry!"

I shared my Small Change, Big Impact™ philosophy with her and told her to do one thing...**eat breakfast.** That's all we talked about during our first visit. I didn't care what time she ate lunch or whether she had veggies for dinner. She had one assignment...to eat breakfast.

We chose a couple of options. She decided she could manage a smoothie or, on some mornings, it would be a yogurt and a piece of fruit.

The next time we met, Kathy said she loved the smoothie and it was a hit with her kids too. After seven days of eating breakfast every morning, her body signaled her to eat about every four hours. She responded with healthy choices and portions that suited her appetite.

By the end of the first week she had the energy to start exercising. Two weeks after our first meeting she was doing a moderate thirty-minute workout on the elliptical four days a week. If she felt hungry after dinner, she would choose fruit or yogurt but most nights opted out and went to bed early. During this time she was menstruating and reported no PMS cravings, which had been something she'd battled with for years.

Remember, I did not tell her to start exercising. I did not tell her what to eat for lunch. I did not tell her to avoid sugar. I just told her to eat breakfast.

In doing so, she gave her body the signal to start burning fuel efficiently in the morning, which prompted the harmonious orchestration of her body throughout the day. Within two weeks she lost four pounds, saying it was the first time she'd been below 140 pounds since before the birth of her first child.

Think of it this way: You will spend $50 to fill up your tank and often drive completely out of your way to make sure you have gas in your car. You do this because you know the repercussions if you don't.

Why, then, would you not make time every morning – in fact, less time than it takes to fill up your tank – to put fuel in your body? Value your machine! Because whether you're four or forty, you can relate to this question:

Do you want to be a fast car or a slow car? A Ferrari or a an old beat-up VW Bus?

Regardless of what those cars look like, you know how they perform.

Choose optimal performance! Start today and Always Eat Breakfast!

Daily Lesson #5:
END OLD LIFE-PATTERNS
WITH A FOOD DIARY

Ah, yes…the dreaded task of writing down everything you eat so that you or some other judging individual can note your dietary pitfalls. Too much sugar, not enough vegetables, and way too much food on your plate.

May you never think this about the Food Diary again!

The reality behind a Food Diary is that it works. Not only will you identify hidden habits and patterns around you and food, you will lose twice as much weight as people who don't keep a Food Diary.

Yep, that's right, and the research proves it.

According to a study by the Kaiser Permanente Center for Health Research, participants who kept food diaries lost almost double the weight of their non-journaling counterparts.

The study, published in the *American Journal of Preventive Medicine* focused on the efficacy of various behavioral weight-loss interventions in more than 1500 overweight and obese adults.

After five months, the participants in the study lost an average of thirteen pounds. However, those who used a Food Diary lost up to twenty-six pounds and they kept the weight off.

Why is this?

Other experts and I agree that the ultimate value of the Food Diary lies in the personal accountability. When you are writing down what you eat, you gain ownership of the choices you make. This ownership gives you an uncommon power around your food choices. You will begin to feel in control of your body, your mind, and your future. This in turn will trigger your innate desire to choose wisely. It's basic psychology.

Dr. Patrick O'Neil, director of the Weight Management Center at the Medical University of South Carolina, says, "Most of us don't really know how much we eat and drink; we have very charitable memories."

I concur with Dr. O'Neil and see how my clients can quickly forget what they eat. When I ask them to report an average day of what they eat and drink, most of them describe healthy diets that include plenty of fruit, vegetables, lean protein, and salads.

So I say, "Wow, this sounds like a pretty good diet. How do you think I can best help you?"

They then reply that they can't lose weight, they feel terrible, and they are confused about what they are doing wrong.

When I start to probe, I find that the healthy breakfast of yogurt and fruit also includes three cups of coffee loaded with sugar and cream. The healthy lunch of grilled chicken includes half a basket of bread and a trip to the office candy bowl an hour later. The healthy dinner of protein and veggies also includes three beers, a handful of chips, and a mound of ice cream before bed.

Sound familiar?

My clients are not blatantly lying about what they eat. Some may hide the truth a bit, but most of them are just unaware – so unaware that the snacks, drinks, and desserts seem like non-events or just minor diversions.

Once I get my clients to track what they eat, they see the truth. The Food Diary becomes a mandatory tool to find the hidden patterns and get results. I can look at someone's diary and notice that every time they eat a fudge bar, it is ten o'clock at night, they're exhausted, and they feel defeated by their day.

With this information, I can effectively coach them to go to bed at nine – before they reach total exhaustion. I can also make suggestions for improving their sleep and counsel them on how to better cope with stress. It doesn't take long before they realize the fudge bar is not the answer.

Do you see how this can be beneficial? The Food Diary, quite simply, helps me to help you.

But here's the catch.

The Food Diary is helpful only when you decide to do it.

In my experience, most people decide NOT to keep a Food Diary. They tell me it's a hassle or that they don't want to face what they're eating every day. I honor that this is partly true, but it's not the REAL reason.

The real reason you don't comply with keeping a Food Diary is because your Fat Kid Mentality is saying, "Don't tell me what to do!" **Deep down, you are being governed by a rebellious nature that's shouting, "You can't make me!" Sadly, this rebelliousness keeps you stuck and overweight.**

Are you with me?

Now, this doesn't make you a bad person. All of us have this rebellious nature on some level. Some of you are even proud of how your stubbornness has served you in positive ways; marching to your own drum can lead to things like starting a business, heading an organization, or warding off the bullies.

But if the reason you don't want to keep a Food Diary is because you don't want to be told what to do, then this behavior has become a limitation that dictates your food choices and your current state of health.

You are stuck in a habitual pattern.

Just like a child who doesn't want to do what he's told, you start to blame your weight on factors outside yourself, such as people, diets, and circumstances. From this place, you will get the results of an undisciplined child and not the results available for you when you surrender and do the work of keeping a Food Diary.

Consider this: Whatever you are resisting about keeping the Food Diary is exactly what you need to face and conquer in order to achieve a healthy weight.

I'll say that again.

Whatever you are resisting about keeping the Food Diary is exactly what you need to face and conquer in order to achieve a healthy weight.

Please allow me to explain.

Remember in Chapter Two when we talked about your set patterns and how they keep you stuck in old ways of Being? These set patterns aren't just isolated to specific events. These patterns show up in all areas of your life.

To be specific, if you are resisting keeping a Food Diary because you don't want to be told what to do, then you resist making sales calls, you ignore requests made by your spouse, you don't follow the speed limit, and you make up your own rules.

Do you see the inherent risk here? Most likely this rebellious nature is affecting every area of your life and you aren't getting the results you want anywhere.

Now here's where you can have a profound shift.

Underneath the rebellious nature lies a feeling. This is the feeling that arises when you are told what to do. You may not know what the feeling is yet, but when you do (by completing the Small Change below) you will have the tools to DISSOLVE the patterns that have been controlling your behavior.

You will break through the Fat Kid Mentality that says, "Don't tell me what to do!"

You will then become hyper-aware of the same patterns playing out in your food choices. If you are making up your own rules in other areas of your life, you're making up your own rules around food.

This exercise will open you up to a new way of thinking about food that will change the way you eat for the rest of your life.

SMALL CHANGE:

I want you to first pay attention to the feelings coming up, right now, when I say,

"You need to keep a Food Diary."

Do you feel excited, inspired, or empowered? If so, that's wonderful.

For those who are experiencing anger, fear, guilt, or some other negative feeling, this is also wonderful! You know why?

Because if you are present to what you are feeling right now, in this moment, then you have identified the very feeling that shows up when you are told what to do. This will also show up every time you make an entry in your Food Diary. And it is THIS feeling that is keeping you fat.

What you are feeling about the Food Diary is what you feel every time you are faced with an event that you perceive as negative. The actions that follow are what keep you stuck in your old ways.

The exercise below will get you present to these feelings so that you can see them for what they are – just feelings. When you do this you can make new decisions around the way you eat and live your life.

1) Describe the FIRST feeling that comes up when I say, "You need to keep a Food Diary." (e.g., anger, fear, resentment)

_____

_____

_____

2) Think back to the first time you felt this feeling (probably in childhood). Write down what was happening and who was there.

_____

_____

_____

3) Now, write down what you do in other areas of your life when this feeling comes up. (For example, if you are feeling anger, what do you do when you feel angry with your husband or significant other? Do you get manipulative? Then this is how you will approach your Food Diary when you feel angry. You will manipulate the guidelines rather than following them as suggested.)

_____

_____

_____

Do you see how this feeling of anger (or whatever it is for you) has nothing to do with the Food Diary? Do you see how this has more to do with an experience from the past that you've carried forward to develop your Fat Kid Mentality and a habitual way of Being?

To let this pattern go, let's come up with your own empowering statement that will reprogram your brain and transform this habitual pattern of rebellion. For example, you could say:

"I agree to commit to the Food Diary NOW because it is the best tool I have to get me to my desired weight."

In doing this exercise and creating an empowering statement, you will set yourself free from your negative beliefs around the Food Diary. You allow the Food Diary to be a powerful catalyst in letting go of the behaviors that dictate your food choices.

You can then use the same method to make new statements around your actual food choices.

For example, you could state:

"I realize my urge to _____ (eat a candy bar, drink glasses of wine, etc.) is just my habitual way of saying, 'Don't tell me what to do.' I know I will benefit from letting others help me."

"I know that when I choose fruit instead of chips, I am following the rules of nutrition that help me live a better life."

"I know that it is my body's natural state to crave healthy food, so I'm pushing my rebellious side out of the way to listen to what my body needs."

Read your statements at the start of every day. They become especially helpful when you're in the throes of your rebellion and need help disengaging from the past and getting present to what you want for your life now.

Once you have completed this exercise, you can get started on your Food Diary.

Please refer to Appendix A for a Food Diary template to use for your journaling.

When you track your food every day, you will have a road map to share with a nutritionist or doctor who can guide you towards healthier choices.

You will also get present to your habits. You may see that you mindlessly snack at the office. Or that you eat chips every day when you thought it was just twice a week. You'll realize you're skipping breakfast and drinking three cups of coffee. Or you may see that you make healthy choices by eating vegetables every night.

The biggest payoff to keeping a Food Diary is that you learn how to end old patterns. You can then apply this to all areas of your life and will start to make choices that bring forth your highest good.

You will then see yourself as the open-minded, vibrant, sexy, confident, fit, powerful, gorgeous person that you are! Here's how keeping a Food Diary changed the life of one of my clients.

BIG IMPACT:

Dennis detested the Food Diary. From our very first meeting, he made it clear that he was not going to log his daily food intake. Nor did he see the value of tracking the patterns related to his food choices. He was a self-proclaimed "emotional eater," so he believed he just needed to get rid of the stress and then he would be fine.

The trouble with Dennis was that he never dealt with the stress. So week after week he would come into my office with the same story about how he had to have the ice cream to deal with his stress. Or that he had to have the martini because he was out with colleagues and was feeling stressed. There was always an excuse.

One day he said to me, "I know, I know, I shouldn't be doing this if I want to lose weight. But I know why I do it, so I guess that's half the battle, right?"

I responded, "Yes, Dennis, this will be a continuous battle. But it's not half the battle – it IS the battle that you face every day, in every aspect of your life. If you want to be free of this battle, then you will commit to the Food Diary and get real with your patterns of rebellion."

He looked at me and then stared down at his hands, shaking his head. When he looked up again, he wore a sheepish grin and said, "Okay, you win. Tell me what to do."

I sent him forth with the Small Change assignment listed above. But before he left my office, we discovered together that the resounding feeling of SHAME came up every time I asked him to keep a Food Diary.

So he went to work to discover when he first felt the feeling of shame. He described a time in childhood when his dad had scolded him for making a bad play on the baseball field. This really embarrassed Dennis in front of his teammates. But the real feeling that stuck was not the embarrassment, but that he had let down his dad.

He felt ashamed for disappointing his dad. And now when he feels he disappoints people, he feels shame. So in this exercise, he revealed that somehow, in keeping the diary, he would do it wrong. So rather than feeling the shame of this, he would make up his own rules so that he could be in control and do it right.

When Dennis discovered how he was attaching shame to something as simple as logging his food, he finally saw the solution for change.

He became very aware that in placing shame onto the diary, he was controlling the amount of coaching I could provide him. He was sabotaging our efforts by keeping me away from the truth of what was keeping him stuck. This is the rebellious nature at work.

He then started to see how his feelings of shame were playing out in other areas of his life. When there was the perceived risk of letting down his boss, he would avoid projects that could have earned him a raise. When he felt that he might let down his wife, he would avoid the intimacy that would create a delicious and lasting marriage.

Dennis then started to see how the feelings of shame kept him from making good food choices. What if he couldn't keep it up? What if he didn't like the food? What if he got really fit and had to go to different restaurants than his buddies?

Rather than feel the shame of letting people down, he stood firmly in his old ways of Being – in the world of rebellion, ice cream, and martinis!

Once he completed the exercise, he realized that his shame from the past was keeping him from being a healthy, fit, powerful, and wonderfully successful man in the present. In this moment, the feelings that were holding him back began to dissolve.

That's not to say the feelings of shame never came up again. But Dennis was able to move through the feelings for the purpose of completing his Food Diary. This then became a powerful tool in getting him to his goal.

It's the same with you. When you use the Food Diary to identify patterns that come up in your life, you will successfully address these patterns, which always leads to better choices.

That year Dennis lost forty-seven pounds. He still has ice cream and martinis every now and then, but he no longer feels shame. He continues to fill the bulk of his day with healthy living practices like eating fresh fruit and vegetables and getting some kind of exercise.

You can do this too.

By doing the exercise above and keeping a Food Diary, you will move through the Fat Kid Mentality of rebellion and shame that keeps you stuck. This, my friends, will move you beyond your limitations, and set you up to succeed in weight, in health, and in life.

BALANCE YOUR PLATE

In the eighties, carbs were good and fat was bad.

In the nineties, protein was good and carbs were bad.

Today, carbs are good (but not the "bad" carbs), protein is good (but not too much), and fat is suddenly a health food (but only if it's "good" fat).

Confused? I don't blame you.

With each decade, experts profess a different point of view. It's no wonder you want to bury your head in the sand and go back to losing weight the old fashioned way – by drastically cutting calories and overly increasing your exercise.

But let me remind you – that didn't work the last time. And it doesn't work for the many other people who rely on cutting calories and increasing exercise as their only method to lose weight.

The myth that we've been taught for decades is that if you eat less and exercise more, then you have a deficit at the end of the day and the pounds will just melt off.

Why is it, then, that when you cut calories and increase your exercise, you still can't lose weight? Or you lose SOME weight, but not the amount you'd LIKE to lose. And do you find it takes much longer now to lose ten pounds? Better yet, how much of the weight are you actually keeping off?

As we discussed in previous chapters, it's not about finding the perfect diet or exhausting yourself with exercise.

Rather, it's about giving your body what it needs!

And what it needs is BALANCE.

If you ignore this rule, and maintain the myopic view of dieting, then you are setting up your body to fail. In other words, your habits and patterns around losing weight will always defeat you, because there is a gap, a missing piece that up until now has never been factored.

The missing piece is a well-tuned metabolism.

Cutting calories and increasing exercise works only when your metabolism is balanced.

Most likely, your metabolism is not well-tuned due to years of stress, yo-yo dieting, high-carb this, low-fat that, and other failed plans. It's not because diets don't work for you that you haven't lost the weight. That's just a convenient excuse. **It's because your body is out of balance, and an out-of-balance body produces out-of-balance results.**

Think of this way.

Take a well-tuned car. You push the gas pedal and your car goes. You press the brake and it stops. Since you take good care of your car – filling it with gasoline and providing proper maintenance – you are sure it will respond to the proper signals.

How frustrating would it be to push the gas pedal and instead of going, your car stops?

You'd be so confused.

That's what's going on in your body when your metabolism is out of whack…total confusion!

An example of this is with my client Jennifer, a twenty-five-year-old woman who came to my office with one question: "What's going on? I'm working out for an hour seven days a week, eating no fat and hardly any carbs, but I can't get rid of these twenty pounds!"

From my expertise, I knew exactly what was going on. The years of over-exercise and cutting out primary food groups – like fat and carbohydrates – was confusing the heck out of her body.

So like the confused car – gas pedal, stop, brake pedal, go – Jennifer's body was slowing down with exercise and dieting, rather than working efficiently to produce her desired results.

Despite my diagnosis, Jennifer was completely dismayed, and, quite frankly, ticked off! It wasn't like she was sitting at home eating bon-bons all day. She was committed, mindful of her diet, and working her butt off at the gym.

So what *was* going on?

I said to Jennifer, "I see that you're frustrated, and I get it. There is a solution. But you need to hang with me for a minute, because what I'm about to tell you is going to dismantle every belief you've ever had about weight loss. I'm going to challenge you to do things you're not going to like."

Jennifer sat back in her chair and crossed her arms at her chest. I could see this was going to be hard for her to hear.

So I asked, "Can you agree to listen with an open mind?"

Sigh..."Yes," she said, "I know I'm here for a reason."

"Okay then," I continued, "here's the deal. You need to eat more carbs, eat more fat, and spend less time at the gym."

Total silence.

But I knew this was coming. She wasn't the first frustrated client who'd heard this advice from me before. I encounter situations like Jennifer's all the time, and the results are always the same. If you exercise too hard, and you cut out the necessary nutrients that your body needs to function, then it will start producing opposite results...weight gain instead of weight loss.

So now not only was Jennifer frustrated, she was also scared to death. In her mind, and quite possibly in yours, the thought of eating more carbs and fat and spending less time at the gym means *gaining* twenty pounds, not losing them.

Am I right?

If you've been living in the world of dieting, and miserably exercising your brains out, you can relate to Jennifer's fear. In this world, the Fat Kid Mentality says, "Losing weight involves frustration and deprivation."

To Jennifer, the thought of allowing herself anything other than this way of thinking, meant giving up and accepting failure.

But here's the reality.

If you've dieted according to one of these failed plans, then you most likely have depleted your body of the necessary nutrients for growth and a balanced metabolism. By depriving your body of the nutrients it needs, you have effectively caused your metabolism to shift. Now your body will not respond to fewer calories and more exercise. In fact, your body is confused and is just like the car with the mixed up signals.

Gas pedal, stop. Brake pedal, go.

Once Jennifer agreed to continue the conversation, I said, "Allow me to ease your fear. Trust me. We are going to radically shift your physiology, and you will lose those stubborn pounds that have kept you stuck in the world of dieting."

"Okay Julie. That makes sense," she said. "But let me get this straight: Are you saying that everything I've been doing is wrong?"

"Not necessarily," I answered. "You do need to be mindful of what you eat and how much you exercise, but there's missing a piece." So I continued to explain.

Despite Jennifer's valiant efforts, she was disconnected from her body. She was approaching weight loss with her mind, believing that her dieting system worked. But what she failed to do was listen to the signals from her body, telling her that the system was flawed. Rather, she kept trying to force her body to adapt to the Fat Kid Mentality that said, "Work harder!"

But being healthy doesn't work this way. The only system that works for your body is balance. So when your diet is out of balance, then your body will follow suit.

When you operate from your habitual programming of dieting and deprivation, you disconnect from your body as a whole. You stop paying attention to signals because your mind is calling the shots. You discount your body shouting out its dietary needs.

For example, when Jennifer was hungry and was naturally drawn to carbohydrates, she didn't listen. Instead she followed her plan of "eat more protein." When her body said, "I need rest," she instead went for a hard workout at the gym.

Your body is clear about what it needs, but you continue to force your plan on it hoping it will change. This is dishonoring your body. You and your body are at war.

Think of an embryo. It knows exactly what it needs from the womb for development and survival. It does not have a voice, but it has an intelligence that works seamlessly with the messages sent to the mother's brain. These messages will then determine things like the mother's hunger cues and her food choices.

For example, when the embryo needs calcium for bones, the mother will crave calcium-rich foods. When tissue is being formed, the mother will crave protein (which can come from vegetarian sources as well as non-vegetarian). When both the embryo and the mother need more energy, the mother will crave carbohydrates.

From my experience, women are most in tune with their body when they are pregnant. This is nature's way of saying, "You must listen and respond!"

Plain and simple, your body knows what it needs. If you choose to listen, it will guide you through your dietary choices with ease.

Are you on board?

Great! So let's talk about how you can get your metabolism back in balance.

The food you eat supplies much more than just fuel for your body. It provides the materials that form your skin, hair, muscle, bone, and all other tissues. Your diet also provides nutrients to manufacture hormones and make brain chemicals that regulate how you think and feel.

When you think about it, if you need nutrients from food to function, what happens when you start to eliminate certain food groups in an effort to cut calories?

The result is that you instruct your body to make up for those deficiencies, and that's where your body will go to war for itself and fight for balance. If you're not eating carbohydrates, your body will retaliate by stealing stored glucose (or glycogen) from other areas of your body – i.e., your muscles. Then you lose muscle mass, so your body responds to that deficiency, and the vicious cycle continues. One depleted area feeds off another...and another...then another.

You really are what you eat and that's why a balanced diet – or in this conversation, a Balanced Plate – is so important.

A Balanced Plate means a balanced metabolism.

So let's divide your Balanced Plate into three primary food groups: Carbohydrates, Protein, and Fat. These are called macro-nutrients. With macro meaning "large," these are the nutrients that your body needs in the largest amounts in the form of calories. This is where you get your fuel.

CARBOHYDRATES

Carbohydrates have gotten a bad rap.

These are foods such as breads, grains, cereals, fruits, fruit juices, starchy vegetables, legumes, sugary foods, some milk products, and alcohol.

But as you can see from the list, not all carbohydrates are bad. Whole grains, fruits, vegetables, legumes, are wonderfully natural sources of carbohydrates. Yet too often they get lumped into the same category as sugary cereals, fruit juices, and candy.

When I explained this to Jennifer, she said, "I've been avoiding carrots and potatoes and nearly all fruit because I thought all carbs were going to make me fat!" At the same time she admitted this would set her up for cravings and then splurge with a Snicker's bar or double margarita.

Now in reality, does it make sense to cut out carrots and bananas, when in the same day you'll eat five Hershey's kisses?

I know you don't see the sense in this, but it's how you've been trained to see carbohydrates in the Fat Kid Mentality.

So when you shift your belief system away from dieting and more onto foods that support a healthy metabolism, you will focus on wholesome carbohydrates that bring balance back to your body.

These sources of carbohydrates are those that come from the earth. You either pick them from a tree or pull them from the ground. They are loaded with fiber and necessary nutrients and are designed (by nature) to serve as your body's **primary source of fuel.**

However, foods that are high in **_refined carbohydrates or sugars_** should be moderated or avoided. It's not as though you'll never have a glass of wine or a piece of birthday cake again. THAT is the dieting and Fat Kid Mentality that we want to break through.

But it's good to know that these higher sugar carbohydrates cause a sharp rise in blood sugar and insulin levels. Over time this can lead to insulin resistance, fat storage, low energy levels, and increased risk of chronic disease.

At the same time, if you cut out ALL carbohydrates – especially the healthy ones – you deplete your body of the essential nutrients that:

- Provide the brain with fuel to orchestrate your body's functions.
- Regulate mood and sleep by building healthy neurotransmitters.
- Provide energy that maintains proper metabolism.
- Slow digestion through high-fiber foods that promote a healthy blood sugar and insulin response.

Most importantly, cutting out carbs starves your BRAIN, which uses about 20 percent of the energy provided by this food group. So when you cut out carbs, your brain will respond by stealing stored energy from your muscles. As a result, you lose muscle mass and slow down your metabolism.

This is exactly how it was playing out with Jennifer. She was cutting out carbs, starving her brain, losing muscle mass, and slowing down her metabolism.

No amount of dieting or exercise was going to get results when her out-of-balance body was winning the battle.

Can you relate to how this dieting cycle has failed you?

Jennifer sure did.

Jennifer realized she needed to embrace the healthiest forms of carbohydrates and learn to eat from a Balanced Plate.

A Balanced Plate means a balanced body.

PROTEIN

Protein is a critical component to many body functions, not the least of which is to stimulate the production of glucagon. Glucagon is a hormone that opposes insulin and stimulates fat-burning in the body. If you want to feel good and lose or maintain weight, it is essential that you eat adequate amounts of protein.

In addition, protein is also important for:
- Growth (especially important for children, teens, and pregnant women).
- Supporting healthy immune functions.
- Making essential hormones and enzymes involved in digestion, metabolism, and tissue repair.
- Preserving lean muscle mass.

But remember, you don't have to eat a slab of steak to get your protein.

This is where Jennifer was getting into trouble. She was afraid of carbohydrates, but getting a little too friendly with protein, mostly because she was so hungry due to her restricted low-carb diet.

At meal times she was eating 6 to 8 ounces of grilled chicken or steak, which was double the amount that her body could actually utilize. In fact, most people only need 3 ounces of animal protein per meal, which is about the size of a deck of cards. An average-sized chicken breast is about 8 ounces of protein.

When you eat too much protein at a meal, your body can't metabolize it in one sitting. If the body can't use food, it stores it. Plus, too much protein taxes your adrenals and can raise stress hormones like cortisol, which also tell your body to store fat.

So we first discovered that Jennifer was cutting out carbs, starving her brain, losing muscle mass, and slowing down her metabolism.

Now we were addressing the fact that she was eating too much protein and raising her stress hormones, which in turn encouraged fat storage.

In her efforts to lose weight with dieting and exercise, she was losing muscle and gaining fat!

To reverse this, just know that small, regulated amounts of protein throughout the day will help to regulate your blood sugar, retain muscle mass, make you feel more satiated, and keep your body in balance. I'll give you some examples of healthy protein sources later in the chapter.

A Balanced Plate means a balanced body.

FAT

Eat too much fat, get fat. Right?

Yes and no. If you eat too much fat, you can quickly add calories to your diet that put you over your suggested daily intake. But just like carbs and protein, certain types of fat are critical to a healthy metabolism. Thus, cutting out fats completely can set you up for a host of imbalances.

We need fat for:

- Normal growth and development.
- A concentrated source of energy.
- Absorbing important fat-soluble vitamins like A, D, E, and K and carotenoids.
- Providing cushioning for the organs.
- Maintaining cell membranes.
- Providing taste, consistency, and stability to foods.

Furthermore, "nonfat" does not always equate with "healthy."

If a food is naturally nonfat, such as a piece of fruit, then that is considered healthy. But if you're like Jennifer, walking down the aisles looking for nonfat labels on salad dressings, chips, yogurt, and EVERYTHING, then you are setting yourself up for disaster.

Here's what I mean.

First of all, when you look at foods for what they DON'T have – e.g., fat – rather than what they DO have – e.g., vitamins and minerals – you are automatically buying into a deadly dieting myth:

That exclusion is better than inclusion.

Now just think about that statement for a moment. **Exclusion is better than inclusion.** If you apply this belief to other areas of your life – relationships for instance – do you think you will experience abundance with friends, colleagues, or even your soul mate?

Probably not.

But when it comes to losing weight, this is the paradigm that resides over your choices. You come from a place of *excluding* things that you think are bad for you, rather than *including* things that are inherently good for you.

Here's an example of how this plays out in your food choices.

You have come to believe that a nonfat salad dressing is supposed to go on top of a bed of greens. If you look at the label on your favorite nonfat dressing, you'll see that the very first ingredient is sugar, usually in the form of high-fructose corn syrup.

So here you have this fresh bed of greens and veggies, and you're pouring sugar on top of it in an effort to reduce fat. Do you think you're body is going to appreciate that you are eating less fat and replacing it with sugar?

Yes, you are cutting out a few calories – about 45 – because there's no fat, but you've actually reduced the nutritional value of the salad because you're drenching it in sugar.

If you had chosen a LOW-FAT dressing made from healthy fats like canola or olive oil, then those 45 calories from the fat would at least be utilized in the body in a way that would restore balance. And remember, when your body is balanced, it burns fat.

So in essence, when you eat the sugary salad dressing on the greens, you're giving your body the raw materials to gain weight. Or, you could choose the salad dressing with healthy fat and put those 45 calories to good use to help you lose weight.

And to add insult to injury, typically the nonfat foods leave you feeling hungry and dissatisfied, which leads to cravings for unhealthy fats and/or sweets.

Now I also understand you may just be confused. You've heard nonfat foods are good for you. So naturally, in an effort to lose weight, you seek out all the nonfat foods.

But it's more about distinguishing fats. You've heard of "good fats" – things like olive oil, Omega 3 oils from fish and flax, and other healthy fats that come from foods like walnuts and avocado. These fats are from the earth and were put on the planet to support optimal human function.

A Balanced Plate means a balanced body.

SUMMARY

So you see, each macronutrient serves a very definitive purpose in your body. **To eliminate one of them puts you at risk for depleting your body of the building blocks it needs to secure balance and overall wellness.**

When you eat from a Balanced Plate with healthy carbohydrates, lean sources of protein, and moderate amounts of healthy fats, your body starts to operate the way it was designed – to maintain perfect weight and perfect function.

Just like a well-tuned car.

Gas pedal, go. Brake pedal, stop.

Here's how you can Balance Your Plate to recalibrate your body and get it back into balance.

SMALL CHANGE:

When you Balance Your Plate and include foods from the three groups of macronutrients, your body will **function in the normal and healthy range. Then your weight will fall into a normal and healthy range as well.**

Let me show you the system to easily integrate this into your daily life.

Believe me, it's much easier than you think. And, the big impact results are totally worth the small changes you'll put in on the front end. I've helped countless people follow this system and it has completely transformed their lives. My clients notice quickly that they have more energy, fewer cravings, better sleep, and improved overall health – not to mention weight loss that sticks!

Here's how you do it:

CARBOHYDRATES

Every meal and snack should contain at least two sources of carbohydrates for quick energy. It's best to choose foods that are lower on the glycemic index – which is a rating of how quickly foods get turned to sugar in the body. The more fiber a food contains, the lower it will be on the glycemic index, so the less impact it will have on your blood sugar.

I divide carbohydrates into two categories to make it easier for my clients:

1) Starchy Carbs – found in grain-based products
2) Produce Carbs – found in fruits and vegetables.

Both of these naturally contain more fiber and have fewer calories than the refined carbohydrates found in white bread, white rice, white pasta, etc.

Examples of Starchy Carbs, and average serving sizes (this will vary based on your body frame, weight, and activity level) include

·   1 cup cooked rolled oats

- 1 piece whole-grain toast
- 1 cup cooked brown rice
- 1 cup cooked quinoa (keen-wa)
- 1 cup cooked whole-wheat pasta
- 5 whole-grain crackers
- ½ whole-grain pita bread
- 1 small whole-grain tortilla

My general rule is that when you choose from the Starchy Carbs, you should have no more than one serving per meal. For example, if you know you're going to have oatmeal for breakfast, then skip the toast. If you're having pasta for dinner, then skip the bread.

This way, you give your body a good amount of complex carbohydrates for slow-burning energy, without overloading the system with more glucose than your body can handle in one sitting. When your body is not equipped to utilize this glucose – due to lack of exercise or an out-of-balance metabolism – then this glucose is more readily stored as fat.

You can also use this Starchy Carb as an allowance for an alcoholic beverage or your favorite cookie or piece of dark chocolate. So, if you plan to enjoy a glass of wine for dinner, then skip the bread, pasta, and/or brown rice that you would have normally had in that meal. Keep your meal to a lean source of protein (see list below), a half plate of vegetables and the wine (or possibly the cookie or Starchy Carb of your choice).

Voila…that's where the magic of the Balanced Plate supports your life choices with EASE. When you diet, you check out on life and deprive yourself of the pleasures that are naturally part of your culture or your environment. The Balanced Plate gives you the power to choose what feels right for you in that moment.

Here's another trick.

You'll be incredibly successful at balancing your metabolism if the majority of your carbohydrates come from fruit and vegetables. In fact, half your Balanced Plate should be filled with a variety of fresh produce. Although some fruits and vegetables may have the same impact on your blood sugar as a piece of bread, produce has the added benefit of vitamins and minerals that are not found in your grain-based choices.

Ideally, focus on fruits and vegetables that are lower on the glycemic index.

Examples and serving sizes include:

- 1 cup blueberries
- 1 medium apple
- ½ cantaloupe
- 2 cups raw spinach
- 1 ½ cups cooked zucchini
- ½ banana
- 1 cup unsweetened applesauce

That's not to say you shouldn't eat the entire rainbow of produce. Just know that the more tropical fruits – papaya, mango, and kiwi – and the starchier vegetables – yams, butternut squash, and potatoes – are higher on the glycemic index and should be eaten in half-cup portions.

PROTEIN

When you hear protein, you think meat. That can be a turn-off to some people or a green light for others to eat the 24-ounce Porterhouse.

Finding a balance with protein, and what's right for your body, is what we're aiming for. There are plenty of lean and healthy sources of protein that can be easily integrated into ANY diet – even vegetarian or vegan.

Ideally men want to shoot for about 25 grams of protein per meal, whereas women want to aim for close to15 grams per meal. Examples include:

- · 1 cup edamame (soy beans) (22 g)
- · 1 cup cooked quinoa with 1 ounce almonds (16 g)
- · 2 eggs (12 g)
- · 2 ounces low-fat cheese (12 g)
- · 4 ounces salmon (25 g)
- · 4 ounces tofu (20 g)
- · 2 tablespoon peanut butter (8 g)
- · 1 cup navy beans (20 g)

See Appendix B for a full list of protein sources and grams per serving.

FAT

Be conscious of adding a small serving of fat to every meal.

Examples of healthy fats and serving sizes include:

- olive oil – 1 to 2 teaspoons per serving
- walnuts – 12 per serving – for a snack, in oatmeal, or on salads
- avocado – ¼ medium – high in calories but loaded with goodness!
- peanut butter – 2 tablespoons – almond butter is good too
- Salba® grain – 1 tablespoon per day – rich in Omega 3's

You want to be on the look out for the less optimal fats.

Some foods are higher in saturated fats, and those are okay as long as you're also cutting back on sugar. If you don't already have high cholesterol or hypertension, and you are relatively active, then a couple times a week you can afford the saturated fat and dietary cholesterol found in whole eggs and lowfat dairy products. I also allow small amounts of butter for flavor – about one teaspoon is fine as a condiment.

What you want to avoid are the **hydrogenated or trans fats** found in commercially prepared foods, such as cookies, cakes, cereal bars, and crackers.

Basically these fats are derived from a liquid vegetable or corn oil (the ones that are nearly void of nutrients) and are put through a chemical process that turns the liquid into a solid. This solid form of fat is then added to foods to ensure a longer shelf life.

These trans fats add no nutritional value to food. Period. And when eaten as part of a daily diet, they are *known* to increase your risk of heart disease and cancer.

So cut out the trans fats and moderate all the healthy fats.

When you factor healthy fats into your Balanced Plate, you will find that a little bit goes a long way in bringing balance back to your body. Watch your portions, and you'll find that you feel better, you feel fuller longer, your hair and nails will be stronger, your hormones will start to regulate, and you will bring a new sense of enjoyment to your wonderfully fresh plate of greens with veggies!

See Appendix C for Balanced Plate Meal and Snack Ideas.

BIG IMPACT:

Well, Jennifer got it.

During one of our conversations she was chuckling, but also a bit teary-eyed when she said, "I feel like I owe my body an apology. Here I am pushing against it and all I needed to do was listen to it."

She also got very present to the power of the body's wisdom. It became very clear that the perfectly crafted systems in the body have their own intelligence. And this intelligence always wins, no matter how much you think you can outsmart it.

If you can let go of your control and open up all the channels for the body to operate smoothly, you will find a sense of liberation that finally frees you from the Fat Kid Mentality that says, "Something's wrong here."

This is where Jennifer had an even bigger shift that allowed her to move away from her old ways and embrace my system of balancing her plate to balance her metabolism.

She finally forgave herself for restricting her diet and over-exercising. She realized that when she was caught in this trap, she just thought she was doing what she was supposed to do.

No one had ever told her to do it any differently! No one held a space for her to appreciate her body's inherent wisdom. No one ever pointed out the *direct* relationship between the food and the function it serves for her body (and every living creature, for that matter). No one ever allowed her to trust the symbiotic relationship between food and optimal health.

No one ever taught her the common sense of the Balanced Plate.

When I told Jennifer she was just misinformed, she felt liberated. She was able to free herself of the guilt around "doing it wrong." In reality, she just didn't know any better. She was bouncing from diet to diet, trying to find the right fix and trusting each new approach because someone else said it would work.

So you might be thinking, "Well, how do I know in ten years the Balanced Plate isn't just another diet-plan-gone-bad?"

You will know when you start implementing it. Because, in truth there is balance, and in balance there is truth. And I've seen it with hundreds of clients who have lost weight, shifted their metabolism, and created lifelong healthy habits just by following the Balanced Plate concepts.

Now it was time for Jennifer to apply her new knowledge. She was responsible for listening to her body. By doing so, she would honor her metabolism's unique requirements through a daily commitment to a Balanced Plate.

She agreed. Jennifer's Balanced Plate now looks like this:

Breakfast:
1 cup cooked oatmeal (starchy carb)
2 tablespoons walnuts (fat)
½ cup blueberries (produce carb)
½ cup Greek yogurt (protein)

Or sometimes it might be:

1 piece of whole grain toast (starchy carb)
2 scrambled eggs (protein w/some saturated fat from egg yolks)
1 peach or other fresh fruit (produce carb)

She also explored some of my smoothie recipes (see Appendix

D) that included protein powder, fruit, and ground Salba®.

Lunch and dinner may look like:

A green salad topped with grilled protein – tofu or some sort of fish – with beans and grilled veggies.

Sometimes she adds avocado or she'll sprinkle some nuts and seeds on it to add a little crunch and some healthy fat. Other times she'll opt for half a hummus and veggie wrap and an apple, or if she's in a rush she'll just have some celery or carrots with almond butter and a couple pieces of string cheese.

She enjoys a cold beer with her boyfriend on the weekends and allows herself a sweet treat of homemade sorbet or a naturally sweetened oatmeal or peanut butter cookie every now and then.

Since moderating her protein and adding more carbohydrates to her diet, she now feels more balanced and just naturally opts out of the bread on the table and skips the white rice at her favorite Asian fast food restaurant.

Before, Jennifer would have felt this was a sacrifice. Now, her body craves the balance of the healthier options, so she really makes these choices without giving it much thought.

After six months of the Balanced Plate approach, Jennifer lost fifteen pounds. Rather than being disappointed that she didn't lose the full twenty pounds, she chose to accept that her body was guiding her to the proper weight that was going to keep her in balance.

We also worked on Jennifer's exercise program and incorporated more diversity in the form of yoga, Pilates, and trail running. This better suited her body as exercise became a celebration rather than a chore. I'll talk more about finding the right kind of exercise for your body in a later Daily Lesson.

Until then, use Jennifer's story to give you permission to accept all the life-giving macronutrients and begin creating a balanced metabolism with a Balanced Plate today.

* Go to www.salbasmart.com for more nutritional information on Salba® and to make a direct order. This grain is rich is Omega 3 fatty acids and fiber which helps to lower cholesterol and triglycerides. It is a perfect addition to any diet and is shown to help with appetite control.

TAKE A TWO-WEEK
SUGAR HOLIDAY

The alarm clock goes off and you hit snooze. It goes off ten minutes later and now you have just enough time to shower, get dressed, feed the kids, make lunches, drive to school, stop for a to-go latte and a sugar-coated doughnut, fight traffic, scramble for parking, and arrive at the office for your eight o'clock meeting.

You are in meetings until two o'clock, grab a carb-loaded lunch at your desk (or skip lunch all together), then rush the kids to soccer, grab greasy fast food on the way home, have a glass of wine (or two), start laundry, read e-mails, take a sleep-aid, have some ice cream, go to bed, and the next day…

…do it all over again.

Sound familiar? You are not alone.

This is "A Day in the Life" of most Americans. It's a clear indication of why fast-paced societies battle with an epidemic called obesity.

But that's not all. This lifestyle creates the cause and effect for conditions like depression, anxiety, and addiction. Of course, we have medications for all of these. And in many cases, this is the required course of care so that people can function in their every day lives.

Then again, maybe not.

You may be someone who's taking anti-depressants, appetite suppressants, or anti-anxiety medications, and it's possible you don't really need them. Often proper nutrition and a shift in your mindset serve to address core issues and eliminate symptoms. I've had several clients who have completely eliminated the need for medications. If you are taking medications now, I encourage you to view them as temporary relief rather than a permanent solution.

Regardless of whether or not you are taking medications, you have adopted unhealthy patterns that are setting the stage for "dis"ease.

What if you were to step back a few paces and look at how your style of living is dictating your life?

Let me say that again. **Your STYLE of LIVING is dictating your LIFE.**

Remember in Chapter Two how we talked about your patterns? You have set patterns of thinking and behaving that shape your reality. As in the example above, the alarm clock goes off and your day plays out the same way from mild insanity to total chaos. And you believe this is just the way it is.

Think of it this way. These patterns are like your body's hard drive. Your body is programmed to respond to external and internal cues. When it receives a cue it responds by performing a specific function. Just like a computer, when you push a certain button, you get a predictable response.

I know this well. This is how my STYLE of LIVING dictated my life.

By the time I was fifteen I had habituated my response to feelings of anxiety and sadness. I would treat these feelings with food.

When I ate ice cream, I felt at ease. When I drank a Diet Coke, I felt energized and in control. As I got older and was exposed to other "stimulants," I found that wine made me feel relaxed and powerful. Cigarettes made me feel content and brave. Stress made me feel accomplished.

All of these substances were my attempt to self-medicate. They gave me a holiday from the constant chatter and the Fat Kid Mentality that said, "You are fat and unlovable." I believed sugar, caffeine, alcohol, and stress were the perfect fix.

It wasn't until I became a nutritionist that I realized how my self-medicating habits had cemented a reliance on these substances for many years. They were an integral part of my life. *They were my lifestyle.*

What about you?

What is your lifestyle? The definition of lifestyle is "the way of life that is typical of a person." Your lifestyle is your **WAY OF LIFE**. It is the way you live day, after day, after day, after day.

This way of life is shaped by your Fat Kid Mentality that says, "I eat when I'm stressed. That's just the way it is. That is my way of life."

Or

"I hate to sweat, so I just don't exercise. That's just me."

Or

"I'm not someone who likes vegetables. I never have been, and I never will be."

How does this way of life feel to you? Is this acceptable?

Do you feel good justifying that you eat when you're stressed? Are you ready to face obesity and disease because you've convinced yourself that sweating is bad? Do you feel empowered when you boastfully state that you won't protect your health by eating vegetables?

Possibly it's something different for you.

Are you unable to function without that latte in the morning? Are you one who migrates to the office candy jar by 10 am? Do you need a three o'clock cigarette break? Are you convinced that you can't sleep at night without your evening cocktail or popping a pill?

Once you have identified how these beliefs shape your way of life, you can start to see the consistent patterns that play out in your body.

You see, all of these "stimulants" – caffeine, sugar, nicotine, alcohol, and drugs – have an effect on your neurotransmitters – chemical messengers that transmit "thoughts" from one cell to the next, allowing brain cells to talk to each other. What's most fascinating is that how you experience emotion is dictated by certain neurotransmitters.

One such neurotransmitter you might be familiar with – serotonin. This is a hormonal neurotransmitter that promotes and improves sleep, improves self esteem, relieves depression, diminishes cravings, and prevents agitated depression and worrying.

Now, keep in mind, there are natural ways to build serotonin that do not include caffeine, sugar, nicotine, drugs, or alcohol. I'll explain more on that later.

First, I want you to think about something.

Imagine the power something has over you when its primary function is to **make you feel happy.** We all want to feel happy, and we want to feel happy NOW. So the reason you like things like caffeine, sugar, nicotine, drugs, and alcohol is because they cue the body to secrete neurotransmitters with such force that you get an immediate high. Perfect!

Now, here's the downside.

This high lasts only for a short time. In reality, your body doesn't like to be in a state of overwhelm. Just like your computer's hard drive has protective measures to keep it from getting overloaded and shutting down, your brain will shut down the body's response to serotonin to keep it from going into overdrive.

You might be thinking, "Cool, I can take all these stimulants and my body will make sure they don't hurt me." That's partially true. But if that were the case, we wouldn't be having this discussion.

In reality, as soon as your body shuts down the production of neurotransmitters, a vicious cycle starts. I call it the **Crave Cycle.** Here's how it works:

When your serotonin is low, you will crave the stimulants that get you high. For example, sugar. You ingest the sugar, and your serotonin increases. Abundant serotonin makes you feel euphoric. Yeah! Then the body senses overwhelm. It shuts off the receptor sites to serotonin so that your body can't use the hormone anymore. Then you feel low again. Yuck. This is when you feel depressed and hear the Fat Kid Mentality that says, "You are fat and unlovable." As an antidote to these low feelings, the body sends out the message, "Give me what you gave me to feel happy – NOW!"

Welcome to your **CRAVINGS.**

I think you know what happens next. You listen to the body's cues and ingest the sugar, caffeine, alcohol, nicotine, and/or drugs. Once again, you feel euphoric. Yeah. And the cycle continues.

A pretty powerful momentum!

Not to mention the effect your habits have on hormones such as cortisol, insulin, and a host of others that regulate your body's ability to burn fat.

These are incredibly intelligent chemicals designed to reinstate balance. Yet the body can't sustain balance when its hard drive has been programmed to cycle between overwhelm and deficiency.

So, you're probably asking, "How do I stop the cycle?"

Simple. You reprogram the hard drive.

If you keep listening to the current messages your body is sending, you will continue to enforce them. Just like with your computer, if you keep pushing the letter "B" on your keyboard, the letter "B" will show up on your screen. If you don't want the letter "B" to show up when you push the letter "B," then you need to reprogram the hard drive.

If you *listen to the body's programmed responses to the low feelings that say,* "You can't start your day without coffee," then you'll drink the coffee with the belief that you can't start your day without it. If it says, "You can't unwind without a glass of wine," then you'll drink wine every night with the belief that you can't unwind without it. And if the message says, "A meal isn't complete without dessert," then you will never walk away from a meal without having dessert.

So again, the key here is to reprogram the brain by rewriting the messages.

The best way to do this is to take away the content that the brain is responding to. So when I say, "Take a Two-Week Sugar Holiday," I'm also referring to the other stimulants – or the content – be it caffeine, alcohol, tobacco, or drugs.

If you are not giving the body the opportunity to respond to these stimulants, it will start to respond to healthier replacements. As I hinted earlier, there are natural replacements that powerfully build serotonin – things like whole grains, frutis and vegetables, exercise, yoga, deep breathing, and meditation. These are the natural stimulants that **also** impact the pleasure centers of the brain.

Now keep in mind that the body will always opt for the quick fix. Remember, we want to be happy and we want to be happy NOW!

The natural serotonin enhancers may take longer to produce results. You may feel frustrated with the wait. But if you hang in there you will see that these natural enhancers create a more sustainable flow of serotonin that will quite literally knock out your cravings – for the rest of your life. Let me take that back. It will knock out your cravings for the harmful stimulants, and your body will instead crave things like whole grains, exercise, deep breathing, and meditation!

Isn't that great news?

It's similar to ending a romantic relationship. When you break up, there is the possibility that someday you can be friends with that person. You can get over him, and then revisit the idea of having him in your life again. Yet you know for now that you can't really get over that person if he keeps hanging around. You've got to create space.

It's the same with stimulants. Sometimes you just need a break.

You also know that some people you just can't have in your life. Period. You break up, and that's it...you never see them again.

It's the same with the stimulants.

The reprogramming won't happen unless you completely "break up." If you say, "I just won't have sugar on Mondays and Wednesdays" or "I'll drink only on the weekends," this won't work. Once your body experiences the stimulant, it will opt for that instead of the healthier "relationships" you have created with the natural serotonin enhancers.

Do you really get that?

While the healthier habits may take longer to create the response you desire, they are designed to give you more energy, more clarity, and more sustainable power.

Once you have successfully avoided the stimulants and feel you do not need them to function, you can ultimately be friends with some of them again. This then allows you to enjoy them every now and then, namely sugar, caffeine, and heart-healthy red wine. (I do not propose letting tobacco and drugs back in.)

Possibly you can invite some of the "friends" over for a special occasion, where you can politely ask them to leave if they become a problem. If you find that these "friends" are just too toxic, then you have the choice to dismiss them from your life knowing they create an unhealthy addiction.

For me, I can enjoy sugar in the occasional dessert or ice cream cone and not be compelled to eat it again for another month. Cigarettes? One puff and I'd be hooked. Alcohol? I opt not to drink it, only because it makes me tired and unclear.

This shift happened for me after taking the two-week holiday from these stimulants and replacing them with healthier, more sustainable options – things like brown rice, protein at every meal, running, meditation, music, fruit, starchy vegetables, and positive thinking.

You will have your individual experience with this. You may be fine with sugar but know you need to quit alcohol all together. Caffeine may be tolerable in green tea, but coffee sets off a whole host of cravings.

You can decide how your patterns will play out. But for now… take the two-week holiday.

Here's how:

SMALL CHANGE:

1) Remove the offender from your home – whether its sugar, cigarettes, or that opened bottle of wine in the fridge. Toss it out!

2) Remove the offender from your work environment – if the bowl of candy sits right outside your door, kindly ask if it can be moved to another location. If not, then find another route so you don't have to walk by the candy bowl twenty times a day.

3) Inform your friends and family of your commitment to taking a two-week holiday from the "culprit." That way, if you choose to opt out of dessert, happy hour, or the 3 pm coffee break, they know what you're up to and can help keep you accountable.

4) Offer to bring your own salad dressings or other condiments, sauces, etc., to parties or BBQs. Again, if you tell people what your mean nutritionist wants you to do, they'll be more likely to support you rather than mock you.

5) Read labels. Sugar is hidden in many of your favorite foods – things like yogurt, crackers, and bread – and can be labeled as cane sugar, maltitol, and high fructose corn syrup.

6) Remember, chocolate has caffeine too so avoid it if trying to cut out the artificial buzz.

7) Sweeteners are synonymous with sugar in my book. The zero-calorie sweeteners send the same message to your brain, "Something sweet is coming in," and promote the same cravings as sugar. Even natural sweeteners like honey and agave nectar, are still sweet and should be avoided for your two-week holiday.

8) If you take a two-week holiday from coffee or caffeinated beverages, do it slowly. Quitting cold turkey is too hard on your body and will set you up for internal stressors. Cut your normal intake by one-fourth every day, so that by Day Four you have eliminated it. If you experience headaches or fatigue on day four try to work through it. If you can't, then hang out with your lowest dose of coffee for another day or two until you can cut it out completely.

9) Replace stimulants with other natural serotonin enhancers.

Here are a few:

· Starchy vegetables such as squash, baked potatoes, and yams offer complex carbohydrates that naturally increase serotonin and provide slow-burning fuel for sustained energy.

· Include two daily servings of high-fiber grains such as brown rice, rolled oats, barley soup, and quinoa (keen-wa) salad. (See Appendix D for recipes.) If you eliminate these grains from your diet completely – as in high-protein, low-carb plans – you are starving your brain from the nutrients it needs to produce serotonin.

· Nuts, seeds, bananas, turkey, tuna, soy beans, dairy products, and eggs are high in the amino acid tryptophan, which actually helps make serotonin. These are best eaten before bed to promote sleep, especially if you've been craving alcohol at night.

BIG IMPACT:

Sandy, a client who repeatedly complained of her addiction to sugar, walked into my office frustrated and resigned. She knew the daily sugar fixes kept her from losing weight, but more importantly, she was a highly paid, successful lawyer and could not understand how a food substance could control her when she was used to winning huge legal disputes.

She could win in the courtroom but not in the trials around her addiction to sugar.

Defeat, however, was not her motivation. She had been to her doctor and the blood work indicated Metabolic Syndrome, presented as high blood pressure, high cholesterol, high blood sugar, and belly fat. If left unchecked, she could end up with diabetes. She is happily married with two small children, so illness was not an option.

Despite her resistance and her glaring looks (although aimed at me jokingly and lovingly), she agreed to my advice of "Take a

Two-Week Sugar Holiday." For two solid weeks, she did not touch sugar. Not only did she avoid the obvious sources, like cookies, candy, and cake, she also vigilantly read labels to make sure she was not getting added sugars in sauces, condiments, dressings, marinades, and beverages.

For the first four days she cursed me. I didn't see her, but I was really hoping I did not break some sort of law that would put me in front of her in the courtroom. She would have had me locked up for sure!

All joking aside, she was successful. She stayed away from sugar for two weeks and completely ended all cravings that had haunted her for years. In doing so, she realized she had power over sugar and broke through her Fat Kid Mentality that said, "I am happy only when I eat sugar."

For so long she had given into the idea that food had control over her. In regaining her ability to choose, she found she did not need sugar to medicate through her fear, calm her nerves, or to make her feel more comfortable in high-stress situations.

This victory over sugar actually instigated another powerful area in Sandy's life. For the first time in her life she found a profound desire to exercise. She hired a personal trainer who came to her house four days a week at 5:30 am to kick her butt into action. She worked out like crazy and found physical strength and endurance she did not know existed!

Sandy's victory over exercise ignited another interesting area. She also learned to travel smart. While her job kept her on the road for several days at a time, she carried snacks of whole grain crackers and fruit with her on the plane. Even while traveling, she started her day with a healthy breakfast of oatmeal or a high-protein, high-fiber portable breakfast shake. In doing so, she managed her blood sugar and stopped using candy or cookies as a quick pick-me-up.

I continue to see this client intermittently for follow-ups. Sometimes her life circumstances get in the way of her better judgment. Yet when she catches herself, and sees that eating sugar is feeding her addiction, she knows what she needs to do. She remembers it takes two weeks to cut out the sugar, reinstate balance, and eliminate cravings. She hears that voice of mine saying: "Take a Two-Week Sugar Holiday."

She does. And she wins.

So what about you? Are you committed to taking the two-week sugar holiday? If so, choose to begin today and allow your victory over self-medicating with stimulants to ignite the beginning of total health and wellness.

BREAK THROUGH THE
FAKE FOOD PHENOMENA

Sugar-free, fat-free, cholesterol-free. No trans fats, no saturated fat, no fatty fat. Added fiber, added protein, enriched, and nutrient-enhanced.

Take a look at any packaged food label and you'll find a litany of claims designed to make you think these foods are good for you.

Sounds great, right? But what does this really mean?

Let me answer this question by illustrating a comparison.

Take a bushel of apples. What do you find on this packaging? Or how about a bunch of carrots, a head of broccoli, or a bag of grapes? Find anything here?

You don't find any claims, right? You may find a short list of nutrients (even though there are literally thousands of nutrients found in these foods – many more than you could fit on a single package) that the government requires as part of a food label, but there are no messages persuading you of the nutritional value.

You know why?

Because you **already know** these foods are good for you. No one needs to convince you that an apple is nutritious. You don't need any persuading to understand that carrots, grapes, and broccoli should be part of your daily diet. You learned this simple fact as a child, and it is supported by mass media every day (just in case you missed class the day they taught the food pyramid in first grade).

Here's the deal.

Nature doesn't need any propaganda.

Food that is either picked from a tree or pulled from the ground is just plain good for you! No tricks, no gimmicks, no confusion.

So the labeling you've grown accustomed to – which advertises health claims rather than resting on the laurels of inherent nutrition – is feeding into a cultural Fat Kid Mentality that says, "Fake food is okay as long as I lose weight."

I know in your heart you don't believe this. I've mentioned in previous lessons that it's easy to fall into the trap of tribal thinking, which currently says food is healthy if it's "fat-free," "sugar-free," and labeled "diet."

Trust me, you've been misinformed.

In fact, these are the very foods that are making you fat.

When you buy a zero-calorie, sugar-free lemonade, please note that this will make you fatter faster than a few lemons sweetened with honey or a touch of sugar.

When you are convinced that a bag of frozen green beans, slathered in butter and sodium, are good for you because the bag states there are no trans fats, then you have been tricked.

If you believe a 100-calorie pack of cookies is better for you because it has less sugar per serving than a banana, then think again.

And if you are buying the bag of fat-free chips believing that they are healthier because they have fewer calories than a baked potato, then you are deceived by the labeling myths that are crippling your health.

That's because these foods are processed. They are tampered with and manufactured to satisfy palates gone awry. They are designed to support a contemporary way of eating that puts fruits and vegetables at the bottom of the totem pole. All of these factors combined supports a method of food production that enhances flavor through fat and sugar, along with a lifestyle based on convenience and cost, rather than optimal nutrition.

Oddly, this way of thinking and eating *conveniently* supports the Fat Kid Mentality that is making you fat, and it is making you sick.

So what's the answer?

Plain and simple.

Eat. Real. Food.

I like to refer to real food as that which has been *"kissed by the earth."* Eating real food is eating the way nature intended, where you cut out scientifically formulated food and focus on the inherent nutrition found in the plant kingdom.

Fruits, vegetables, nuts, seeds, legumes, and whole grains are all part of this food category.

What is so amazing is that once you start eating real food, you will acclimate your palate and your physiology so that you will start to *enjoy* these foods.

One of the largest world health studies is actually proving this. This multi-year survey is designed to determine what effect adding a whole-food-based nutritional product to the family diet can have on family's health. The study is designed around three interrelated premises:

- Improved nutrition leads to healthier lifestyles and overall better health.
- Good nutrition and other important health habits are best established in childhood.
- Parental support and involvement are the keys to successfully establishing good health habits in children.

Adult and child participants report that over 80 percent of them have become more aware of their health in general and over 90 percent of participants have some positive result to show for it. The study also shows that participants are eating more fruits and vegetables, are reporting fewer sick days, and are taking fewer over-the-counter and prescription medications.

Remarkable results!

Now, let's see what happens when you buy into the labeling myths of processed food.

I refer to processed food as "fake food," because these items are stripped of their nutritional value, **serving only to satisfy taste, hunger, and your need for calories.** They are not designed to provide solid nutrition with the essential nutrients found in whole foods.

Without these vital nutrients, your body will go into a starvation mode. That is because you are *starving* your body of the building blocks it needs to survive. Depriving your body of nutrients is like building a house without the foundation

And here's the real catch.

A starving body will constantly be hungry.

You may ask how you've survived thus far with the processed foods you've been eating. This opens up a critical shift in our conversation from one that centers on mere survival to a more meaningful discussion focusing on life, optimal health, fitness, abundance, vitality, and longevity.

Fake food will keep you alive. And you may or may not live a very long life. The inherent risk is that eating all those chemicals, without the protection of those nutrients found in fruits and vegetables, will lead to disease. So you may live long, but will you live well?

Real food, on the other hand, gives you LIFE.

You can merely survive or you can have life. Life equals energy, power, strength, mental clarity, sexuality, beauty, greatness, prosperity, harmony, laughter, family, opportunity, and sheer joy.

Compelling, don't you think? A little different than the Fat Kid Mentality that keeps you stuck in a world where you spend more time focusing on what NOT to eat, rather than exploring the guilt-free enjoyment of all the foods you CAN eat.

When you eat real food, you provide the nutrients that allow your body to regulate hunger, burn fat, and eliminate cravings. The other profound benefit of eating real food is you increase your desire for other healthy habits, like drinking more water, exercising, and a getting restful sleep.

A starving body never experiences these habits as desires. A starving body simply lacks water, fitness, and restful sleep.

When you starve your body by eating fat-free this and low-cal that, your body cannot do what it was designed to do. You don't have the raw materials from phytonutrients – plant nutrition – that allow your cells to function properly. So your body will be without the essential players to regulate all the systems that keep you in tune.

When you starve your body, you lose the ability to eliminate sweet cravings. You kill off the hunger and full cues that allow you to regulate your portions naturally. You deprive your body of the flavors that actually acclimate your taste buds to fruits, vegetables, grains, and other foods from the earth.

Without a diet rich in real food, you will continue to lose the battle for a healthy body and a healthy weight. The only ones winning are the food manufacturers who keep telling you that fake food is good.

SMALL CHANGE:

The more whole foods you eat, the more your palate will crave these foods. Your body craves what you give it most. Ideally, you should be eating an average of nine servings of fruits and vegetables a day. Athletes and pregnant women should be eating closer to twelve to eighteen servings! This may sound like a daunting number, but with a few adjustments, you'll be hitting that number before you know it.

Try new produce: Instead of sticking with the same five fruits and vegetables you always choose, add one new produce item to your cart every time you go shopping. Vegetables like kale, bok choy, and Swiss chard are often overlooked and can be amazingly delicious additions to your diet. Try this yummy recipe:

SWEET POTATO CAKES WITH KALE

2 cups mashed sweet potatoes or yams
   (I prefer yams with orange flesh)
1 bunch kale, trimmed and sautéed in 1 tablespoon olive oil
1 tablespoon chopped, fresh sage
1 egg white
2 tablespoons ground Salba® seed,
   or whole-wheat bread crumbs
Sea salt and pepper to taste

Preheat oven to 425°. Combine all ingredients in a large mixing bowl. Form into four patties. Lightly grease aluminum foil and place it on top of a cookie sheet. Put patties on top of foil and bake in oven for 30 minutes or until patties are slightly firm. These are also yummy served cold the next day and easy to tote to work, etc.

Incorporate fruits and veggies into every meal: For example, make sure you're eating at least one fruit or veggie with breakfast and lunch, and two with dinner. I have my clients – adults and children – send me a list of ten fruits and ten vegetables they are willing to include as a permanent part of their diet. I take the list and e-mail them ideas for integrating these foods into their diet. Here are some examples:

Fruits

Raspberry – in pancakes or waffles; mixed into plain Greek yogurt or kefir topped with honey; in a bowl topped with milk, soy milk, or cream.

Strawberry – on top of salad greens with poppy seed dressing (1/2 cup canola oil, 1/2 cup water, 1/2 cup honey and 2 teaspoons poppy seeds); on a peanut butter sandwich; dipped in creamy, low-fat cream cheese.

Pineapple – mixed with cottage cheese; as a pizza topping; mixed into coconut milk yogurt; cooked into chicken or tofu stir-fries.

Cranberries – dried cranberries (unsweetened) sprinkled on a salad; dried cranberries (unsweetened) mixed with wasabi peas for a crunchy, sweet snack; in granola and trail mix.

Green grapes – in Waldorf Salad (see recipe); frozen (delicious!).

Olives – make an olive paste by putting olives, olive oil, and sea salt into a food processor and spread on crackers; chopped and mixed into tuna salad: great on their own.

Avocado – yum…half an avocado sprinkled with sea salt; cubed on top of salads; mixed into rice and beans; spread on a tortilla wrap with shredded carrots and lettuce.

Vegetables

Broccoli – as a pizza topping; lightly steamed and topped with butter and sea salt; mixed with olive oil, lemon, salt, and roasted walnuts; Broccoli with Sun-dried Tomatoes (see recipe).

Asparagus – roasted or grilled; cooked, diced, and mixed into pasta sauce; lightly steamed and chilled, then rolled up in a tortilla with honey mustard.

Corn – mixed into black beans and rice; on the cob; cooked and sprinkled on top of salads.

Brussels sprouts – roasted and sprinkled with shaved Parmesan cheese (or cheese of your choice) so that it melts on top; steamed to very soft and then mashed with olive oil and sprinkled with salt and pepper – this is delicious!

Carrots – shredded and added to chicken salad; dipped into hummus or guacamole; in Minestrone Soup (see recipe); made into Carrot Pattie (see recipe).

Lettuce – use in place of tortillas for yummy wraps (e.g., turkey, grilled chicken, cheese); put in sandwiches every chance you get; add a salad to every meal, especially when you eat out.

Potato – homemade fries; baked and topped with cottage cheese or salsa or guacamole; red potatoes boiled, chilled, and dipped into your favorite salad dressing or hummus.

Cucumbers – on salads; as a sandwich: peel cucumbers, slice thin, and put on whole-grain bread with a little Italian dressing and sea salt (one of our family favorites for picnics, although when we were little we loved this on white bread :); Cucumber Salad (see recipe).

Artichokes – yum…my son Max loves these grilled; put artichoke hearts on top of pizzas and salads; Healthy Artichoke Dip (see recipe).

Edamame – lightly steamed with sea salt; put beans on salads; great snack!

Build meals around vegetables: There are a hundred recipes that use vegetables as the main course. Homemade veggies burgers, stir-fries, and gourmet salads all use veggies as their main component. This is not to say you need to be a vegetarian. It is simply my recommendation to explore new ways of eating vegetables by making them a main course.

Incorporate fruits and vegetables into all of your recipes: Chop produce into most recipes for an added boost. For example, grated carrots into turkey burgers, shredded cabbage into soups, chopped zucchini into pasta sauce.

Understand serving sizes: A serving of fruit or vegetables is 1-2 cups depending on your size. A real easy way to remember what is right for you is to use your fist as a guide. If your portions match your clenched fist (including fingers), then you're doing great. But remember, you really can never eat too many leafy greens and other non-starchy vegetables.

Prepare food ahead a time: If you don't feel you have the time to prepare a whole food meal every night, set aside a few hours during the week dedicated to making meals that can then be frozen and eaten in a hurry later in the week.

Make it fun: Make introducing more whole foods into your diet an enjoyable experience by picking your own fresh produce from local farms that offer "pick your own" services. Or hire a nutritionist to take you to the grocery store to explore the produce aisle and come up with new creations for your menu. (Contact us at www. juliehammerstein.com to locate one in your area.)

Explore Farmers' Markets: Spend a Saturday exploring your local farmers' market for the freshest and most delicious produce available. The farmers are very passionate about their crops and will take extra time to offer cooking suggestions.

Whole Food Concentrates: When you just can't eat your total servings of fruits and vegetables – whether due to time or financial constraints – then please consider a whole food concentrate. Whole food concentrates take fruits and vegetables, render them into a powder, and deliver them in capsule or chewable form so that you can get all the benefits of the phytonutrients in a cost-effective and convenient form. The most effective and safe products will have the following:

1) Primary research – peer-reviewed, double-blind, and placebo controlled, showing the health benefits of the product itself, not just a component of the product.

2) All natural ingredients without processed fillers, sweeteners, or artificial coloring and flavoring.

3) Approval by the FDA to be sold as a "food" rather than a supplement, which is not controlled by the FDA.

BIG IMPACT:

My client Pam was stuck on fake food.

She proudly proclaimed hating vegetables (except for lettuce) and admitted to liking fruit, but only apples, strawberries, and tangerines. She said bananas scared her because they had too much sugar, and she stayed away from potatoes because they were too starchy and she liked them only with butter, sour cream, and bacon bits.

She drank three Diet Cokes every day, chewed sugarless gum to stave off hunger, and doctored her coffee with nonfat creamer and the powdery stuff in the pink, yellow, and blue packets. She ate sugar-free yogurt, snacked on fat-free chips, and lunched on low-sodium, low-calorie frozen meals. For dessert she'd fill up on sugar-free, low calorie ice cream, after having eaten her standby dinner of low-fat cheese, popcorn, and lettuce with fat-free Italian dressing.

She worked eighty-hour weeks, wasn't exercising, and her idea of drinking water was the one glass she got at night when she downed her handful of nutritional supplements.

Pam was tired, she was hungry…and she was fat.

She had gained forty pounds over a five-year period and was tired of spending her days ruminating about food. Her fridge was bare, but her cabinets were stocked with packaged foods that supported her life of dieting.

Pam was also scared, because all she knew was fake food. She grew up eating diet food because that's what her mother ate. And it served Pam well during her teens and twenties, where much of her focus was on staying skinny.

Pam couldn't figure out why she was gaining weight around her middle and, at just thirty-five years old, was feeling achy when she got out of bed and caught every virus that came her way. She was constantly craving sugar and fat and couldn't stand the idea of one more high-protein, low-carb, energy bar.

Thank goodness Pam was a good sport! When she was describing her habits to me, it was as if she was doing a stand-up comedy routine, openly hazing herself and laughing at the insanity of her food choices. She had me in stitches when she described hearing the soundtrack to Jaws every time she entered the periphery of the grocery store…you know, the area where all the fresh food resides?

With that admission, I knew Pam was ready for change and was going to be a willing participant in the plan I had for her – a plan that included a balanced plate, focusing on small amounts of lean protein and healthy fats (as described in Daily Lesson #6), and TONS of fruit, vegetables, and whole grains.

I also knew that I had to meet Pam where she was and take her where she needed to go. I needed to bridge the gap – or the deep abyss, in this case – between what Pam needed to do (eat real food) and what she was actually doing. She was capable of eating more healthfully, but it was a large space to fill, having spent her entire life in the world of fake food.

I started her on whole food based nutrition, including a juice powder concentrate from 17 different fruits, vegetables and grains. Each ingredient is specially selected to provide a broad range of nutritional benefits. I explained to Pam that this was not a substitute for fruits and vegetables, but something that could augment her diet so that she could achieve the 7-9 servings of fruits and vegetables that I recommend to all my women clients. (Men require 9-12 servings of fruits and vegetables per day).

The food concentrate, called JuicePlus+®, was going to offer Pam much better outcomes than the handfuls of vitamin supplements she was taking, which were causing her stomach upset and putting her further into the Fat Kid Mentality that supported fake food. Pam believed that she could keep doing what she was doing, and her vitamins would protect her.

What she didn't realize is that her body was still starving for synergy – the natural coming together, so to speak, of nutrition that is found in REAL FOOD. The JuicePlus+® naturally serves as a catalyst for the body to want real food, to better assimilate and absorb real food, and to continually send messages that it is thriving on real food.

Pam loved the idea that she could get some easy solutions to her problems. I loved the idea that she was getting whole food based nutrition that was going to radically retrain her brain and transform her physiology.

Within four months, our program did just that.

We devoted one of our sessions to looking back at the previous four months to measure her progress. We had made an itemized list of things she wanted to accomplish, and we started to check off the completed goals. It looked like this:

1) Eat more fruits and vegetables – Check. Pam was drinking a fruit smoothie every morning and had expanded her vegetable intake to one vegetable at night, such as zucchini, sweet potatoes, spinach salad, and grated carrots.

2) Drink more water – Check. Pam was down to one Diet Coke per week (remember, it used to be three per day) and had set her phone alarm to notify her to drink a glass of water every hour. She was successful most days.

3) Eat fewer artificial sweeteners – Check. Pam had not used a pink, yellow, or blue packet in four months! She sweetened her tea, oatmeal, and plain yogurt with honey and cut down on her foods with fake sugar. She was still eating the sugar-free ice cream at night, but that was it.

4) Do more cooking at home – Check. Pam was rotating seven different recipes I'd given her that focused on whole grains, olive oil, lean protein, and tons of vegetables. I also gave her some ideas for baking to get her acquainted with wholesome treats that did not come packaged on a shelf. She actually baked me some cookies with real sugar, whole wheat, oats, walnuts, butter, raisins, soy milk, and eggs. They were delicious and Pam admitted to enjoying them in moderation.

5) Exercise more frequently – Check. Pam was experiencing more energy, so she was able to get up early two mornings during the week to fit in a twenty-minute workout before work. We were still working on this goal, but this was a start that Pam relates directly to eating more real food.

6) Lose forty pounds – Partial Check. In four months Pam had lost twelve pounds. I told her that to lose weight, she had to first correct the imbalances in her body that had occurred while eating all the fake food. She felt frustrated until she noticed all the other benefits that were supporting optimal health. She knew in time that even though she was eating food with more calories, they were more nutrient-dense and for the first time in five years she wasn't starving!

Throughout my professional career, I have never seen shifts in health and client compliance in the way that I do now with whole-food intervention that introduces the body to ***real food.***

I know that Pam was grateful to have found a solution she could commit to every day without feeling like she had to change everything in her diet at once. It was a gradual, yet totally natural process that has become a habit for life – a habit that she enjoys because it has given her back her life in ways that she never imagined.

She enjoys shopping for food now and finds joy in a sale on artichokes. She takes her friends to the farmers' market and makes them dinner out on her patio. Gone are the days of popcorn in front of the TV. She looks forward to parties where she can eat freshly prepared dishes, knowing that she is feeding her body what it needs to self-regulate.

You too can harness the power of real food nutrition. Just small changes of adding more produce into your life every day can manifest huge life changes in your health, your weight, and your well-being.

For more information on JuicePlus+®, please visit www.juiceplus.com.

CREATE A NEW LIFE TEMPLATE

I t's Monday morning.

Today's the day you're going to lose weight and get healthy!

You plan to eat right and exercise, and this time you're committed! No excuses.

You hop out of bed, ready to make it work, and then...

...your life happens.

You realize you haven't allowed time to eat breakfast, so you skip it and grab a latte on the way to work. You are booked with meetings all day, so you miss your planned exercise during the lunch hour. You feel distraught over a conversation with a negative friend, so you ease the stress with a doughnut from the office lounge.

By the time you get home to prepare a healthy dinner for the family, you are exhausted and realize you need to spend two hours

helping your kids with their homework. You order pizza for everyone and eat three pieces because you're starving.

After the kids go to bed, you walk into your home office with
the hope of getting some work done. But your desk is a mess, and
you've misplaced the bill that needs paying this week. You're frustrated and decide you don't have time to prepare the healthy lunch
you wanted to bring to work the next day. You call it a night, vow-
ing to restart your weight loss plan the next day.

It's Tuesday morning.

You wake up to the same life. Nothing has changed – you're
late, you're busy, you're stressed, you're disorganized, you don't
exercise, and you make unhealthy food choices.

Yet in the midst of this you **really do** want to lose weight.

So, what's stopping you?

That's right, it's your Fat Kid Mentality, convincing you that life
is too busy and you don't have a choice. This is just the way life is.

But this is not the way life is. It's just the way YOUR life is. You
can make life look however you want, which is exactly what this
lesson will teach you.

The key to success is to create a "life template" that ensures
your plan to lose weight is congruent with the patterns of your life.

The template of your life is the way you've always done things.
It's a blueprint or a mold with a certain structure that you have
adhered to day after day, year after year, with predictable results.
The very nature of a template is that it's static, and nothing ever
changes.

The problem is that you want things to change. You have all these great intentions, but something keeps getting in the way of you following through on them.

When my clients ask me why this happens, I answer:

"You can't put new goals on an old template."

It's impossible to take a new set of healthy practices – such as exercise, meditation, or healthy meal planning – and integrate them into a life template that is not designed for these activities.

Currently, your life template is set up so that every day you wake up late, skip breakfast, stay disorganized, and so on. If you take NEW goals and try to put them on this OLD template, the system doesn't work. So to successfully integrate the new goals, you need to take specific action steps that allow new habits to fit in.

When I first began to take care of my health, I made several changes to my life template that allowed me to integrate healthy habits, like running, into my daily routine. One of the most important changes I made was to block out every afternoon for exercise. I explained to my friends that I couldn't commit to any plans after school because I needed to reserve this time for exercise. Bringing my friends in on my plan made it much easier to stay on track, because they knew not to tempt me with invitations that would lead me astray.

Rearranging my schedule to allow for running, was not the only change I made. In fact, that was just a small piece to the bigger picture changes that allowed me to really commit to my new life template.

The biggest change I made was to alter my beliefs and my vision around what it meant to be healthy.

I had to shift from the doubt of the Fat Kid Mentality to full-out believing that I AM a healthy person. I had to shift from a state of worry to one of faith. And I had to envision the life I wanted, making sure that I came from a place of pure conviction that being fit and healthy was simply meant to be. And, in fact, once I started to believe that this was possible, I became fit and healthy,

The steps below will show you how to powerfully create your new life template.

SMALL CHANGE:

There are three steps you need to take to create a new life template. Complete these steps, and you will be astounded at how quickly you are able to integrate healthy activities into your life with EASE.

CREATE SPACE

If you want the gift of health, you need to create space in your life to receive it. Just as though someone were to place this gift in your hand, you would need to first let go of what you are holding.

The universe abhors a vacuum. So when there is space, it's Nature's job to fill it. Nature is designed to fill this space with something beneficial. Notice that I said it is "designed" to do this. Now this doesn't always happen, because there are opposing forces – such as negative thoughts or practices – that would attract something unwanted into that space. But if you are really intentional about bringing goodness into your life, then Nature will respond accordingly.

Since Nature is friendly, it will fill it with good. So if you want greater good in your life, you need to make room for it in a new life template and create the thoughts around what you want to come into this space so that it will happen in accordance with

Nature. When things are in accordance with Nature, they happen with more ease.

What can you clear out of your life to create the space that will allow healthy habits to come in?

Let's look at what I call the "time killers." These are unproductive activities that make up your current template and drain your day of energy and time. Once you identify your time killers, you need to eliminate them. At first they may seem insignificant. Yet, when you add them up during the day, you'll see how they consume a considerable amount of your time and mental energy.

These time killers include:

· Unnecessary tidying around the house.

· Watching TV even though you're not interested in the show.

· Searching the Internet rather than sticking to specific Internet-driven tasks.

· Responding to e-mails during the day that can be saved for the evening.

· Gossiping with friends.

· Spending non-strategic time on social networking media.

· Arguing with spouses or children.

· Playing video games.

These are just a few. If you can think of more, take time right now to write them down.

_____

_____

_____

_____

_____

_____

Once you've identified your time killers, STOP DOING THEM! This may seem like a big step to take, so if anything, just eliminate a few and see what happens. If you really want to get present to how these activities are killing your day, start to track how much time you spend doing each. Let's say you spent twenty minutes watching TV, ten minutes needlessly tidying, and fifteen minutes with random Internet searches.

That's forty-five minutes! That's enough time for a workout, to prepare a meal, to write in your Food Diary, or to cut up fresh fruit and vegetables for snacking.

TAKE TEN MINUTES

If you got out of bed ten minutes earlier, what could you get done in that time that would promote healthier habits? Or let's say you tagged on ten minutes at the end of the day by getting rid of your time killers as listed above. What could you get accomplished with this ten-minute change in your life template?

Here are some ideas

· Meditate.
· Take a ten-minute walk around the block.
· Make instant oatmeal and grab a hard-boiled egg for the ride to work.
· Grab a ready-made protein shake or protein bar for breakfast.
· Take your nutritional supplements with a big glass of water.

- Warm up a frozen whole-grain waffle and pair it with string cheese for your kids.
- Stretch or do ten minutes of a yoga video.
- Add ten minutes to your twenty-minute workout video.
- Pack workout clothes for the gym.
- Write in your journal.
- Walk ten more minutes with the dog.
- Read a short story to your child.
- Prepare your child's lunch for the next day.
- Plan the next night's meal.
- Put together your grocery list for the weekend shopping trip.
- Put aside a baggie of healthy snacks (e.g., almonds, fruit, string cheese) to take to work the next day.
- Read ten minutes of a self-improvement book.
- Pick out one, new, healthy recipe and check to see what ingredients you need to buy.
- Cut up some broccoli and stick it in the steamer.
- Throw cooked chicken breast on some packaged salad mix and add cooked garbanzo beans and bottled dressing for an easy dinner.
- Organize your desk or sort through the mail.

You HAVE the time to live healthfully. You just need to create the space for beneficial activities to fit in.

CALL IT IN

Do you know the power in asking?

You have an idea of what you want your life to look like, but you forget to truly ask for what you want in a meaningful way. Whether this be through prayer, through conversation with others, or in a spoken message to the universe, *asking for what you want is a critical first step in getting what you want.*

Perfect health belongs to all of us.

Your desire to be healthy comes from an essential part of you. Your true spirit – hidden under the layers of ego and human experience – knows abundant health as being unequivocally yours.

So often my coaching clients feel uneasy when I ask them to envision their best life. That's because it's unnatural for humans to think beyond a certain idea of what life should look like. I ask them to dream BIG and really imagine what it would feel like to be at their ideal weight. What would it look like if their newfound health inspired them to run a marathon, find a lifelong lover, or generate a seven-figure income?

What about you? Can you imagine?

If you said no, you can't imagine, then this exercise will be very helpful for you. It will help to unleash the possibilities that are dormant, just waiting to be set free and manifested.

If you said yes, then I invite you to expand on your current vision. Make it bigger, grander, UNREASONABLE! Let go of those limitations holding you back and know to your core that what you imagine comes from pure inspiration and your life's purpose.

What do you want your health to look like? I mean, what do you **really** want? If you could wave a magic wand, what miraculous events would take place in your life that would allow for perfect health? Would you absolutely love fresh, wholesome food? Would you run a 10k race? Would you fit into a size 6? Would you invent new, healthy recipes and write a cookbook? Would you be a spokesperson for healthy living?

Sound crazy?

Well, take it from me. I thought so too. But remember, I was the fat girl. I was fifty pounds overweight. I was the one who did the Dieting Dance over and over again. And you know what I'm doing now?

I'm running a 50-mile race in Mexico. I'm wearing designer jeans and tucking in my shirts to show off my waist. I'm craving foods like salmon, broccoli, brown rice, and mango. I am writing this book and living the life of a global advocate for healthy families.

That's because I follow these steps every single day to "call in" exactly what I want out of life. I don't just imagine perfect health, and then shrink it down to fit into reasonable expectations. I ask for exactly what I want, and it shows up in the most amazing ways. Even better, the more I ask and believe in the asking, the faster I receive what I ask for.

You can read more about this in the Big Impact story below. For now, please proceed with this exercise of calling in perfect health.

Write down your top ten desires around your health. Again, these do not need to be reasonable requests. Think of the magic wand and dream big!

1.

2.

3.

4.

5.

6.

7.

8.

9.

10.

Take each desire and describe how it would feel if each one came true. For instance, if your desire is to have tons of energy, how would you feel every day if you had such abundant energy? Or if you could fit into a size 6, how would that make you feel every day?

Now take out a piece of paper or a journal. I want you to write a story about your life that includes all of these desires and feelings as being part of your life. Imagine yourself living into EVERYTHING you listed above. What would your life look like?

You have now created your life for the calling.

It is your responsibility to tune into this vision and ask for your desires to manifest in your life. Whether through prayer, meditation, journaling, or just speaking to a higher source (e.g., the universe), you must consciously ask every day for everything you've listed in your story of perfect health.

This is best done by focusing on daily, monthly, and yearly intentions. But rather than asking for what you want in the form of a request, you want to call it in by stating your desire as something that already exists.

You can use the samples below to guide you.

Daily: Find a time, preferably in the morning, to write your daily statement.

For example: "Today I am enjoying healthy food, and I spend time savoring every bite of my freshly prepared breakfast."

Your turn:

_____

_____

Monthly: At the beginning of each month, you can expect miracles by writing what my business and spiritual coach calls a "monthly surprise" that will show up sometime during the month.

For example: "I love my six-mile run and lose inches around my waist and my thighs. (Rather than "Please let me get up to six miles this month so that I can lose weight.")

Your turn:

_____

_____

Annual: List five to ten desires that you believe will show up in your life over the course of the next 365 days. You can also do this exercise again, if you wish, on the first day of the new year. These are not RESOLUTIONS, which implies that there's a problem to fix or *resolve.* Rather these are intentions or REVOLUTIONS that will *evolve* over the course of the year with solid action steps.

For example:
1. Get to 130 pounds.
2. Buy new wardrobe.
3. Meet life partner.
4. Run the 10k race on Thanksgiving.
5. Collect 100 new recipes I enjoy cooking.

Your turn:

1.

2.

3.

4.

5.

6.

7.

8.

9.

10.

There is so much power in calling in what you see for your life. These aren't just wishes but solid visions of what is going to show up in your life. The key to this is to let go of the idea that these are just fun ideas. Rather, you need to have full-out conviction that one year from now the things you have listed will have ARRIVED!

With this belief, you will be utterly amazed at the miracle of life. Keep reading to see how I changed my life template by following this system.

BIG IMPACT:

I have always had a very strong belief that I will get what I want if I ask for it. I don't say this in a boastful or demanding way, but rather that I believe there is a force greater than I – God, in my case – who has devised a plan that delivers only greatness. So, if I want that greatness to show up in my life, I just need to ask for it to arrive. If I don't ask, then possibly I'm not ready for it.

Even in my darkest hours, when I was miserably overweight and depressed, I knew I would always be taken care of – that somehow I would find a solution that would get me out of an ugly mess. Admittedly, there were times when "being taken care of" meant being rescued. I attracted people who would band-aid a situation so that I could get to the next phase in life, but I wouldn't really learn how to do things differently.

This was never a sustainable solution. Yet I know to my core that I created the space and called in the people and opportunities that got me what I wanted in that particular place and time.

And you know what? You can too.

Even if you don't believe that God or a higher source is the grand deviser of your life, getting what you want by asking will still work. You may believe that you need to ask more of yourself by tapping into an internal force that generally moves you forward in decisions.

You see, I learned much later in life that we all have this power. We are all blessed with the power to create WHATEVER WE WANT in our lives. Those things you call "coincidence" or "circumstance"...you created them. Those things you call "miracles" or "unimaginable"...you created them. The people, situations, opportunities, events – everything that happens in your life – you have made space for and called in.

When I got present to this, I realized I could harness this power for more desirable results and with more ease. Rather than calling in a diet that would offer temporary solutions, I asked for guidance in learning how to listen to what my body really needed. As a result, I was drawn to going back to school to get my training in nutrition and living by the principles I learned through this process.

To this day I am learning how to harness this power and ask for results that are aligned with exactly what I want – no matter how unreasonable they may seem.

For example, rather than trying to find another physical therapist to rehab my knee so that I could train for a marathon, I just created the intention that running would continue to be my exercise of choice, and I would find a way to heal my body and keep running. I called in resources that would show me how to do this by honoring my body.

A few months later I started dating my boyfriend, Andrew. He gave me a book that taught a way of running that's used by the best ultra-marathoners (people who run 100-mile races) in the world. I devoured the book and started trail-running with Andrew shortly thereafter. He also offered some coaching, and within a few weeks I was trail-running thirteen miles with no knee problems.

Rather than beating up my body to train for marathons (which I failed at because I kept pushing something that wasn't meant to be), I am now gracefully training for a 50-mile run in Mexico. I am up to twenty miles, in the mountains, with no problems. I knew I wanted to run, and I get such a high by being out in nature. If I had kept forcing the marathon training, I would have never experienced the exuberance and full-out spiritual experience of my runs with Andrew on the trails just minutes from our home.

You can do this too.

Creating a healthy body and fit life doesn't mean you need to be training for ultra-marathons. All you need to do is envision your perfect scenario and just keep focusing and trusting that vision... every single day! If you do this and stay committed to your vision, I guarantee that something or someone will show up in your life that allows that vision to manifest.

Now, this may not happen tomorrow. In fact, it may take several years for your perfect vision to come true. But as said before, the more conviction and trust that you place on your visions, the faster they become a reality.

It takes practice, but believe me, one day you will write a daily intention and by the end of the day – even sometimes within a few hours – it will come true.

Daily Lesson #10:
CHANGE YOUR IDEA OF REWARD

I have a dear friend who had a heart attack.

He survived, yet several health conditions followed, and now he can barely exercise or engage in life activities without pain. Despite these life-changing events, he continues to drink too much alcohol and binge on high-fat foods. Every night he drinks a bottle of wine, and he spends the weekend eating burgers, fries, and sauce-laden pasta.

He says he "deserves" food and wine, viewing them as "reward." He works hard, he's raised four kids, and he's getting older and doesn't see the need to change his ways.

How could he be so stubborn? Does he not see that his so-called reward is compromising his life? How difficult would it be to choose a different reward? Better yet, why couldn't being successful and having a wonderful family and home life be reward enough?

If you are sensing my feelings of frustration, please know that is the part of me that doesn't want to lose this dear friend to another heart attack.

The nutritionist in me, however, knows that choosing food as your reward is a hard habit to change. It is also common human behavior.

In fact, you all do it as part of your Fat Kid Mentality that says, "I work hard, so I deserve this."

Unarguably, people need to be rewarded and encouraged for their endeavors. To desire a reward is not a bad thing.

The trouble comes when the reward centers on food. When you focus on food as your reward, you naturally justify unhealthy eating habits because you believe they equate to praise. In this detached place of the Fat Kid Mentality, you find less reward in the accomplishment itself and more in how food makes you feel happy, calm, and deserving.

For example, the common conversation is:

"I spent the entire day working on my daughter's school project, so I deserve a glass of wine."

Or...

"I worked out really hard yesterday, so I deserve to go out for a burger."

Or...

"I've lost ten pounds, so I'm rewarding myself with a chocolate milkshake."

While it's great to celebrate, do you see how the actual accomplishment gets diminished in the face of food as the reward? Instead of just BEING with what your actions brought forth, you feel a compelling need for something physical to fill in wherever the external praises left off.

Why is this?

One reason is that you grew up with food as being your reward. Notice, that's the Fat Kid Mentality.

At school, home, and throughout your community you were offered food as a reward for good behavior. Possibly your parents offered you pizza so that you would stop crying. Or you were allowed that piece of pie for finishing your homework or eating your vegetables.

Sound familiar?

You're not alone. Food is a culturally accepted reward. In fact, it's built into the way that food is marketed as an inexpensive and easy way to create positive reinforcement.

But how is food *truly* rewarding you?

Are the handfuls of M & Ms feeling like a reward after your doctor explains that you're at risk for disease? Do your kids benefit from dessert as reward when they're getting teased for being fat?

I know that, in the moment, the reward feels justified. Like my friend, the fries feel like comfort from the stress of a long workweek.

I guarantee, however, that in the moments after his reward, joy is quickly replaced with guilt and blame. Remember the Fat Kid Mentality is built around guilt and blame.

It is my job to make sure that you don't get to this place. I am here not only to show you how to choose a different reward, but also to find equal value in rewards that aren't centered around food. In doing so, you will embrace the natural and healthy rewards that are all around you.

This is not to say you'll never have a glass of champagne or a four-course dinner for a celebration. I'm also not proposing you forgo enjoying a piece of dark chocolate with your spouse because it's delicious. These are all wonderful pleasures in life.

What I'm proposing is that you place more value on rewards that don't have anything to do with food. By doing this, you shift your mindset around food to have it become just a part of daily life, rather than something you need to justify as reward.

In this place, you have the cake because you want the cake, not because you are rewarding yourself for a hard day. You have the glass of wine because you want the glass of wine, not because you are rewarding yourself for being nice to an unruly client.

When you've mindfully created other options for rewards, you open yourself up to a full spectrum of rewards that bring about the same pleasures as food, yet promote healthier outcomes.

The real benefit is that over time your accomplishments will be sufficient reward. No longer will you need outside reinforcement to build self-esteem, calm the mind, or motivate certain behaviors. You may choose to celebrate with the dinner out or the vacation, but they will simply be add-ons to the good feelings you get from having an accomplished day.

SMALL CHANGE:

The first step is to create a new list of rewards.

I know this seems trite. And it's probably not the first time you've been told to do this. Yet, I'm going to show you how to make this more meaningful, so that you will actually use this list not only as your guide, but as your saving grace.

The idea is to create rewards that are *long lasting*. If you are using food as a reward, the good feelings will stop as soon as you finish the meal or the treat. So rather than buying into the old mind-set of immediate gratification, move into big picture thinking that gets you beyond the twenty minutes of joy and into a new realm of healthy living.

It's up to you to choose rewards that support your desires around health and wellness.

If you keep this end-goal in mind, you will find that your rewards have more meaning. You will value them as you get more present to how they produce results that are directly aligned with your desire to be healthy, lean, and fit.

Don't have your rewards counteract the vision you have of being healthy.

For example, if in the past you have rewarded yourself with a movie, only to find that you can't resist the wafting aromas of buttered popcorn, then don't add "going to the movies" to your list of rewards. This is not aligned with your vision.

Now, if you can go to the movie and truly enjoy it without the popcorn, then go to a movie in the middle of the day and enjoy every morsel of a juicy film that motivates and inspires you.

You will actually have two lists. One will be a list of Immediate Rewards, and one will include Future Rewards.

The Immediate Rewards will include things like getting a pedicure or spending an hour at the bookstore. Your Future Rewards may take a few months to acquire, like buying new clothes or treating yourself to a trip with your family.

Keep in mind what I said earlier...if going to the bookstore means you can't pass up the latte and the scone at the bookstore café, then don't put that on your list. Or if planning a trip with your family means going to Disneyworld where all you'll be eating are hot dogs and cotton candy, then plan a different trip.

Remember, it is up to you to choose rewards that support your desires around health and wellness.

Learn to trust your gut about these rewards and what your body and mind truly need as its reward right now. This takes presence of mind! Be present and listen to your body's desires.

For example, my client Sherri would always reward herself with dinners out when she was traveling for work. When she wasn't traveling, she worked long hours from home, and then had to care for two young children at the end of the day.

When she traveled, she really missed her family but felt the need to let loose and enjoy adult time with colleagues. At the same time, she felt a little resentful for being away from the comforts of home.

With her valiant efforts and the sacrifices she made to earn the family's second income, she felt the need to reward herself at the fancy client dinners she attended while traveling.

Sherri realized this would get her off course. At home she could maintain her healthy habits, but she was stuck in the idea of reward equating to expensive wine, five-course meals, and two large lattes every day.

I asked her to come up with her new list of rewards. The first reward on her list was to get a massage. When she read this to me, we both laughed.

We knew that getting a massage wasn't a realistic reward while on the road. Her schedule just didn't allow for it, and she would just be setting herself up for disappointment if she couldn't pull it off. Instead, we thought of what she could do that would meet her needs but also fit into her travel schedule.

In rewriting her list, she said one of her Immediate Rewards would be to buy a small and fun gift either for herself or her kids in every city she traveled to. It wasn't going to be expensive – possibly a small toy, fragrant soap, or a beautiful postcard. We decided she was spending $5 to $10 every day on her lattes, so she could instead transfer this to something that connected her to her family.

This also was in compliance with her health goals, which was to kick her caffeine habit and eat smaller portions. Rather than rewarding herself with food and wine, this new reward helped Sherri feel like traveling could be congruous with who she was at home.

I'll share Sherri's results with you in the Big Impact story below.

Until then, if you're having trouble getting started, here are some examples of rewards you can add to your list:

Immediate Rewards:

1) Light candles and spend twenty minutes alone (in prayer, meditation, or just sitting in silence).
2) Read a book outside in the sunshine or get dirty in your garden.
3) Download music from iTunes and make a favorite CD mix. (After a long week of writing, I reward myself with

music. Burning CDs for my friends keeps me out of the kitchen so that I don't reward myself with a late-night snack.)

4) Close all the shades and take a nap, or go to bed two hours early.

5) Schedule a facial, acupuncture treatment, or just a scalp massage at a local salon or wellness center. (I actually enjoy giving myself pedicures, in silence, maybe with some music playing, after everyone's gone to bed.)

6) Close your home-office door and spend time on the Internet researching hobbies or topics of interest. (Don't get online and look for new recipes – that will just send you into the kitchen.)

7) Schedule a game of golf or a walk in the park with the friend who is your biggest fan and always makes you laugh out loud.

8) Color with your children – it is very therapeutic to color a simple picture.

9) Buy fresh flowers and/or decorate your home for the season (I love to get pumpkins, gourds, and dried leaves from our yard to make a festive centerpiece for the table).

10) Turn off your computer, put on your sweats, and order a movie in your hotel room.

Future Rewards:

1) Take the day off to sit in the park or read magazines by the pool.

2) Plan a romantic trip with your spouse or significant other – this could be a "stay-cation" where you drop the kids at Grandma's and settle in for a weekend of doing nothing at home.

3) Save for that gorgeous piece of jewelry or fabulous pair of boots.

4) Plan a fishing trip or guys/girls weekend in a healthy

environment. (Remember if the fishing trip means beer and baked beans, just be mindful of your goals towards health and wellness and possibly plan something else.)

5) Register for a powerful seminar or speaker and bring a friend or relative.

6) Buy tickets for a play or concert. (After completing my "Max's Minutes" DVD I rewarded myself with tickets to the play *Wicked*. The $100 I spent on this was more aligned with my health goals than spending the same amount on a high-calorie dinner.)

7) Your accomplishments could reward you financially, allowing you to donate to a charity, offer your time for volunteering, or spend more time with family. (My long-term reward with this book is the freedom it affords me to be at home for my son Max.)

8) Aim for fitness rewards like running a marathon, walking a 10K race, joining a hiking club, or getting back into tennis. (Your Immediate Rewards could tie in nicely if you choose to go for a walk that would improve your fitness for your Future Rewards.)

9) Share your success with your friends. Take time to send a letter letting people know of a special recognition you received at work or when you achieved greatness. They will lovingly call you to offer praise and congratulations.

10) Hire a nutritionist to work with your family to come up with meal plans and other tools for success so that the entire family can live healthfully.

BIG IMPACT:

Sherri's list grew as we continued to develop her instincts around healthy rewards.

Once she shifted her focus from food as her reward, she made different meal choices at the dinners out. Rather than grabbing the bread before dinner, she reminded herself that bread was never on her table at home, so she opted out. Rather than drinking two or three glasses of wine, she chose to savor one glass on just one of the nights she was traveling and chose it for the flavor rather than the reward.

As a result, she added exercise to her list of Immediate Rewards and found that giving herself time in the morning to go the hotel gym was a bigger reward than sleeping in from what she described as a "food coma." The reward of exercise then supported her Future Reward of running a 10K race with her girlfriends.

After several months of making these shifts, Sherri came to see me for another follow-up. In our conversation, she realized she no longer needed the rewards as a way to feel okay about her travel schedule.

She accepted her situation as it was and integrated her habits at home into her daily life, regardless of the circumstance. She naturally chose protein and vegetables at dinner and found that eating the bread and having dessert was not a natural choice.

She also found that the feeling she got from exercise *was* the reward. Whenever she finished her morning in the gym she felt energized, happy, confident, and could move into her workday with an ease that she never felt before.

She still missed her family and would often go back to buying small gifts for them just to feel connected. The difference is that she didn't eat huge meals and desserts with the idea of "I deserve this." She knew she was more deserving of the clarity, joy, and freedom that enriched her life through fitness and a healthy weight.

Sherri just felt good about herself, which was a ***huge*** reward. In feeling good about herself, she became acutely aware of how the wine and the overeating was the exact opposite of reward. In fact, she saw how her old ideas of reward totally sabotaged what she now describes as her "clean and inspired living."

Please know that changing your idea of reward doesn't happen overnight. It takes time and conscious effort. Your first step is to sit down and make your list. Keep it in sight. Refer to your list every day. For years I kept my list in my purse on a laminated index card. That way I could read it when I was tempted by rewards that weren't healthy.

Whenever I felt the need to reward myself with a scone or a half bottle of wine, I would consciously pull out my list and find the reward that I could easily transition into – in that moment. No right or wrong, just whatever felt most closely aligned with what I needed in that instant.

Once you come up with your list, and try this out, you'll find that you too can move away from food as your reward and establish joyful practices that keep you aligned with your goals of health and wellness for a lifetime.

NOTICE THE POWER OF SELF-CARE

Do you realize that every time you walk out of the house, you make a statement on how you want the world to see you?

I know you don't think anyone is paying attention, and you're partly right. Some people will take notice of you, and others won't. But that's not the point. The point is that you have a belief about yourself, and you will act a certain way to make sure others see you the same way.

How you want the world to see you dictates the clothes you wear, your hairstyle, the car you drive, what your house looks like, the job you're in, and whom you choose for your significant relationships.

This way of being also plays out in other choices and behaviors, such as the food you eat, the way you talk, the way you walk, how often you get health check-ups, what books you read, how much you exercise, and how much time you spend with other people.

To simplify this a bit, you can see how you present yourself by identifying with one of two statements:

1) "I do care" or 2) "I don't care."

You're going to fall into one of these two categories: You do care about yourself or you don't care about yourself. Either way, you're going to make this statement every time you walk out the door.

Let me paint a picture.

Let's say you take yourself to BE someone who is shy, fat, lazy, and unworthy. With this mindset, do you think you fall into the "I do care" camp or the "I don't care" camp?

From my experience, if you believe you are shy, fat, lazy, and unworthy, then you fall into the "I don't care" camp. Not because you truly don't care, but because if you DO care, then you need to let go of all the negative beliefs you have about yourself. It's much easier to hang on to the beliefs and then get others to believe the same by saying you don't care.

Do you see the trap?

This is the Fat Kid Mentality. This is the mindset that shuts you off from the world by saying, "I don't care, so why should you?"

Here's how that typically looks.

Your appearance is disheveled so as not to draw positive attention from others. You walk slowly and avoid eye contact. You steer clear of social situations, although you don't like hanging out at home because that's where you engage in unhealthy behaviors like overeating or watching too much TV. You are generally tired, which helps justify "that it's just too much trouble" to get up and take a shower before heading out the door in the morning.

Again, the general message is "I don't care, so why should you?" It's very effective. When you send the message that you don't care about yourself, then it's very hard to get others to feel any differently. So in this act of showing the world you don't care, you get the same handed back to you. Yes, you are this powerful. You do get what you ask for!

Now a person who practices self-care generally believes she is worthy of greatness. This person walks out of the house in a very different way. She gives some thought to what she wears. If she decides on workout clothes and a baseball cap, she still presents herself in a positive way. She walks briskly and will be the first to open the door for others or say hello to a stranger. Even if she's just going to the grocery store, she will move with purpose and with confidence.

Here's an interesting observation. Notice the woman who is fifty pounds overweight but still dresses impeccably. Even though she admits to being overweight, do you get the sense by looking at her that she believes herself to be shy, fat, lazy, and unworthy?

Her daily presentation, out in the world, says something very different. And in taking on this presentation of herself, she can move more readily into healthy behaviors such as proper diet, exercise, and self-care. Once she is given proper guidance and the tools unique to her success, this woman will attract healthy behaviors simply by presenting herself to the world as "I do care."

How are you presenting yourself in the world? Is there something you do every morning that puts you in the statement of "I don't' care"?

Little things can send this message. Wearing the same, stained, baggy sweats every day. Forgetting to brush your hair or your teeth. Leaving dirty dishes in the sink or never making your bed. When you ignore these little measures of self-care, you are buying into the Fat Kid Mentality that says to the world, "I don't care, so why should you?"

When you shut out the world, then you are shutting down on yourself. From this place, you will be less inclined to take on life-giving behaviors such as eating a healthy breakfast or getting in a thirty-minute workout.

From the place of "I don't care," you will also shut yourself off from all the greatness that is waiting to come into your life. You won't be open to great romance. You won't allow yourself to join the women at work who walk during lunch. You won't notice the flyer for the cooking class on how to make quick, healthy meals. You won't hear the conversations about books and radio shows geared toward inspiration and personal growth.

In that place of "I don't care," you close yourself off to being anything other than your self-view of shy, fat, lazy, and unworthy.

So how do you shift this? How do you set yourself free from the confines of the "I don't care" Fat Kid Mentality?

You CAN be the full expression of "I do care!" From this place, you will not show the world anything less than total health and wellness. You will naturally start to eat right, exercise, and carry yourself as the vibrant, sexy, yummy, amazing person that lies underneath those baggy sweats and the façade of "I don't care."

You can start right now with little, daily steps of self-care...the things you do every day before leaving the house.

Here's how it works:

SMALL CHANGE:

Today I want you to do identify ONE THING you will do before you leave the house that says to the world "I do care." If you're having a hard time identifying what this is, then think what you would do if you knew that when you left the house you were going to meet the love of your life. Or that when you walked into work your boss would be interviewing you for a promotion. Or that you could run into a friend and be asked to an impromptu dinner.

Would you wear different clothes? Possibly you'd style your hair differently. Maybe you'd put on makeup or rinse and moisturize your face. Maybe you'd shave or wear a certain color shirt. These are single steps you can take to move you into the place of "I do care."

Try this every day for a week, then see what happens. You will be amazed at the transformation. All of a sudden you'll notice more people smiling at you. Or you'll walk at a faster pace and get more accomplished at work. Possibly your children will be happier when they're with you, and friends will call and invite you to go out more often. You may just get that hot date – even if it's with your spouse!

Then you'll start to see an even bigger payoff around healthy eating and exercise. You'll be inspired to eat breakfast, write in your journal, or fit in an early morning workout. These are all the life-giving habits that seem so impossible now but will soon become your way of life.

And what's so magical is that you'll naturally transition out of "I don't care" to "I do care"…with EASE. Not because you're forcing the change, or because I said it would happen, but because *you will genuinely start to care.* You will suddenly place huge importance on who you take yourself to BE and the positive impact of projecting that person out in the world!

Here's how this exercise profoundly changed the life of one of my clients.

BIG IMPACT:

Carly had been my most challenging client for the past month. After years of severe depression, weight gain, food addiction, and pretty much giving up on life, Carly spent most of the time in our weekly meetings trying to unravel the past so that we could focus on her present state of health.

Once we identified what was holding her back, a whole new world opened up and Carly began getting results.

We started by getting her to eat breakfast. This step moved Carly forward, but it was near impossible to get her to commit to the other dietary and exercise changes I created for her program.

I paid close attention to Carly's daily habits. I noticed that every time she came to see me she was very unkempt. Her hair was messy, she hadn't washed off her make-up from the day before, and her clothes were stained and wrinkled. She also complained that her house was a mess, and she didn't like spending time there. Yet she hated going out because she didn't like the way she looked. As a result, she would stay home and binge on candy and huge portions of food.

It was very clear to me that Carly was stuck in the "I don't care, so why should you?" mode. If she didn't care about how she was presenting herself to the world, why would she care about the things she needed to do for herself in the privacy of her home – e.g., eating healthy, exercising, maintaining a clean house, etc.

So one week I decided that her ONLY goal for the next two weeks would be to take a shower every morning and get dressed for the day. She could not leave the house until she had showered and put on clean clothes. I didn't say she had to put on make-up or wear anything fancy, but she had to look and feel as though she would meet her future boyfriend at the coffee shop.

So she did what I suggested. She sent me an e-mail two days before her appointment saying she couldn't wait to share all her good news!

She walked into my office at 3 pm absolutely glowing! She wore an elegant black skirt and a chic, white, button-down blouse. Her hair, clean and shiny, hung gently to her shoulders. She was tan, smiling, and had a playful energy I'd never seen in her before. She told me she was showering every day, going to the coffee shop, and then coming home and eating breakfast. In these two weeks, she also had started walking daily and had made new friends at a book club.

She thanked me profusely and said, "Julie, no one has ever approached weight loss with me like this before. Dieting has always been really overwhelming, and I would get frustrated and quit. But these little steps every week have absolutely changed my life and I'm so motivated and happy."

Better yet, in the weeks following Carly lost twelve pounds and was on the road to physical and emotional recovery. She was feeling so good about herself and her potential that, soon after, she quit eating all forms of sugar and started drinking water instead of diet soda.

Carly continues her journey. She knows that some days will be easier than others. She admits, however, that her best days come when, after waking, she showers, gets dressed, and prepares to receive greatness in her day.

You can do this too with just one small step. Get ready for your day, every day, with the statement "I do care." When you care, others will care, and by the very nature of this attitude, you break through your Fat Kid Mentality and embrace healthy habits as a part of your daily life!

Daily Lesson #12:

BE THE FORCE THAT GETS YOUR BODY IN MOTION

According to my friend and fitness expert, Theresa Byrne, the main reason people don't exercise is because they are afraid they won't "do it right."

This is a valid fear, especially if you believe that by exercising you are entering into a competitive environment where success is measured by how well you do it.

You tell yourself that you don't exercise because it hurts, or it's an inconvenience, or you feel embarrassed by the way you look, or that you don't like to sweat. (Have you convinced yourself of this one?) And these may be true. But the real reason you don't get started is because you believe you won't meet the set standards of exercise – as if there were any.

As a result, you won't try yoga because you aren't flexible enough. You won't run because you're not fast. You won't give kickboxing a shot because you can't kick high enough. You won't take dance because you're not graceful.

Sound familiar?

But who sets the bar? Who dictates what is right or wrong? And who really cares?

You care. You care what people say because, like most of us, you are afraid of being judged. You get caught in the trap of caring what people think. This gets especially tricky when you are accustomed to being good at things. So if you think you will be bad at a certain exercise, you are less likely to try it.

And some of my clients have shared with me that they won't go to the gym until they have lost some weight. Again, they care more about what others will think about them than they care about their fitness goals. Do you see how you can't win with this mentality? You want to lose weight and you can't lose weight without exercise. You won't exercise because you're afraid of what you look like and what others think about what you look like.

In the twelve years that Theresa has coached clients on transforming their mindset around exercise, she has learned that the first step is to give people permission to be a "student" of exercise.

I asked her what she meant by this:

"Look, you're not going to be a professional exerciser, so who cares how well you do it? You just want to be fit, and you are going to have a different starting point than the person next to you. So the trick is to go into it with curiosity and not the expectation that you need to be an expert."

This made so much sense to me. So often I find that my clients are downright fearful of exercise. They have so much trepidation about moving their bodies, simply because they think they will look silly or exercise won't have an impact unless they're sweating hard for sixty minutes on the treadmill.

Exercise is a journey rather than a destination, even a game of sorts. You can go into it with your own set of expectations instead of trying to measure up to what you think is expected of you – all the time remembering *that you're doing it because you know it is what's best for you,* regardless of skill or rate of improvement.

The idea is to move your body. And once you start moving, you will continue to move. Take Newton's First Law of Motion:

"An object in motion will stay in motion and an object at rest will stay at rest unless acted upon by an external force."

The rate at which you move is up to you. Everyone starts at a different place. Remember, I started with just eight blocks. You may choose to start with a ten-minute walk around the park. But believe me, however you choose to begin will be the committed action that changes everything. You choose what feels right to start. Then, if you decide you'd like to achieve results more quickly, you can increase your ten-minute walk to a thirty-minute walk. Do you need to be an expert at walking? Does committing to walking mean that you then need to then commit to running?

It does only if you decide that running is what you'd like to achieve.

And if it is, then be a student. Ask someone for help. Watch what other runners do. Be curious about how to do it. Be open to finding skills you didn't know you had. Be willing to break through thresholds that have held you back – all the time remembering that you are allowed to learn about what is best for you.

When I'm training for long-distance runs, my goal is not to be fast but to be efficient. So, I am a student on how to be more efficient, not a student on how to win the race. If I wanted to win the race, then I would study different aspects of running. It's all up to me.

And what you want to focus on is up to you as well.

Theresa also made this shift in her thoughts about exercise many years ago, and it changed her life. You can read her story below. But first, she coached me on the five steps you can take to become the "force" that gets your body into motion.

SMALL CHANGE:

Identify the First Steps:

Find a Support Coach – This may be a class instructor, a personal trainer, or a friend who is accomplished at the type of exercise you would like to learn. Not only will this coach give you the how-tos, but he or she should be someone who points out your progress, someone who will readily say, "LOOK WHAT YOU HAVE DONE!" And, by the way, this will usually have nothing to do with your weight. Your coach should also have the knowledge to guide you toward new goals, so that you can reach the level of fitness that is aligned with your desired results.

Start With the Positive – Find an exercise that builds on something you already love to do. So, if you love to cook, then walk to the store to get the ingredients for a recipe you are excited about. Or if you are motivated by numbers, then create a spreadsheet so that you can track and check off daily goals. If you love being out in nature, then go for a hike rather than trudging it out on the treadmill. If you like to spend time on your own, then carve out twenty minutes for an in-home yoga video.

Remember, the quantity doesn't matter at first...the *quality* of the activity is what counts.

Prepare for the Dork-Factor – I love how Theresa describes the awkward beginning stages where you fumble around a bit with your newfound exercise. She says that when you start something new, you will feel a bit uncomfortable with the movements for about two weeks, even sometimes up to two months. I can totally relate. I'm taking a karate class with my son right now who is training for his black belt, and I felt very intimidated the first few times. (Yes, even in a class full of seven-year-olds.) Once I decided to embrace the dork-factor, I started having a blast. The ego is gone, and I'm open to what the teacher and the kids teach me.

Focus on the Unexpected – When you really pay attention, the first results you experience will be internal rather than external. This is a critical distinction, because if you don't notice how exercise is affecting you emotionally and mentally, then you will lose sight of why you chose to learn this exercise. You chose it because it was in alignment with what felt right for you. If you then move into a place of judging success based on your pants size, you will develop a resistance to the exercise. You will also build a resistance to yourself and what you're willing to learn. So train yourself to notice the subtleties, like the fact that you're sleeping better, or you have more energy, or that you feel a sense of accomplishment every day. Then all of a sudden you'll see the external results that you wouldn't have noticed, like how your biceps are a little bigger, and your legs are leaner, and your skin is clearer, and your clothes fit better, and so on.

Exercise is a pathway to that internal guide that knows what's best for you. When you follow what's best for you, you achieve your desired physical results.

Listen to Your Body – We are so trained to push through pain. No pain, no gain, right? How's that working for you? Not so good, I bet.

Now that's not to say you shouldn't go beyond a long-standing set point. There's always room to experiment with higher levels of fitness. But notice the difference between someone forcing you into something and your CHOOSING to push yourself. Again, it comes down to paying attention to your body and knowing what feels right. If you've been doing the ten-minute walk around the park, and you get an internal message that says, "This is too easy" or "I wonder if I'm really getting anything from this?"...LISTEN to the message. This is your body giving you the go-ahead to bump it up a notch and seek higher levels of performance. This is very different from listening to an instructor scream at you to get down and do a hundred push-ups when you've never been able to do just one. It is also very different from letting yourself believe that other people are setting the standards. Your body's wisdom will guide you as long as you are willing to pay attention.

BIG IMPACT:

For years Theresa struggled from debilitating chronic fatigue. She was constantly exhausted and could barely move. Doctors and therapists kept telling Theresa that the exhaustion would continue to feed on itself unless she started exercising. This seemed nearly impossible, and she was angry that everyone kept telling her to move her body when she could barely get out of bed.

Just like me when I ran my first eight blocks, Theresa was determined to heal. She started walking around the neighborhood. She would come home exhausted, but the next day, she would get up again and walk the same route again. Over time this turned into longer distances, and she gained courage, strength, and the under-standing that small changes really do make a big impact.

Now Theresa is a third-degree black belt in martial arts, a fitness instructor, personal trainer, motivational speaker, life/empowerment coach, and creator of *Finding Your Voice,* a self-empowerment pro-gram for adults.

After training thousands of kids and adults in the Denver area on how to lead a healthy lifestyle with her martial arts, fitness, and life coaching expertise, she was asked to co-star with me on the TV reality show, *Fitting In*. Her personal success inspired her to help others, which birthed *The Revolution,* a DVD program that gives people the tools and inspiration to lead healthy lives by connecting their mind, body, and spirit.

"It all started with motivation," states Theresa. "Sometimes losing weight is not enough to motivate people. That's when I ask them to look deeper. Possibly they will be motivated to exercise because they want to see their kids grow up. Or because they are tired of breathing hard every time they walk up the stairs. For some, just losing weight to feel more attractive is enough. It's up to you to tap into what drives you."

What you will find is you begin to want to exercise and it won't be a struggle.

"I decided that I could choose my outcomes. I could either struggle or I could just allow things to happen in whatever timeline felt right," Theresa says. "When I knew that I could walk a little farther, I increased it to the level that felt comfortable, all the time listening and learning and choosing to be okay with the process."

Theresa committed to the idea that nothing is "bad," just "interesting." Notice the contrast. When something in her life is interesting, it denotes a sense of curiosity. And in that space of curiosity, she became more open to what exercise could bring forth in her life.

Never in her wildest dreams did Theresa think she'd be a professional athlete. Yet this is where she found her voice and her purpose in life – teaching people how to get fit and live their best life.

Imagine what exercise could create in your life. The possibilities are endless!

You've got to start somewhere. The idea is to just move your body. First find an activity that lights you up, find a coach that inspires you, focus on the positive, and follow your internal guide. And know you don't have to be perfect. Expect the unexpected and be ready to receive the results you desire.

Today you are the force that gets your body in motion. Take it on and you will be surprised at how much joy exercise brings to your life and becomes a big part of who are, not just what you do.

Daily Lesson #13:
PRACTICE GRATITUDE

"Gratitude unlocks the fullness of life. It turns what we have into enough, and more. It turns denial into acceptance, chaos into order, confusion into clarity.... It turns problems into gifts, failures into success, the unexpected into perfect timing, and mistakes into important events." ~ Melody Beattie

I love the simple, yet profound teaching of this quote.

It suggests that **you** have the power to transform the circumstances of your life – the ones you see as negative and out of your control – by changing your perception of these situations.

How do you do that?

You can decide to give thanks.

That's right.

By practicing gratitude for everything that occurs in your life

– and I mean EVERYTHING – you bring forth the desirable from the undesirable, the wanted from the unwanted, the joy from the despair, and the triumph from the defeat.

Sound too easy? Possibly a bit unrealistic?

Allow me to explain.

All too often you limit yourself to feeling grateful when the right conditions or circumstances prevail. You are programmed to believe that when something shows up in your life that you *don't* want – e.g., a flat tire, a breakup, a lost job – that this is bad. Then when something comes around that you *do* want – e.g., a new house, a vacation, a healthy child – this is good and something to be thankful for.

Okay, so we agree on this.

Now let me expand. Remember in previous chapters where I talk about your hard drive? I use this term to refer to the human programming that takes your thoughts and turns them into your reality. If you think something is bad, then it is undoubtedly bad. If you think something is good, then it is undoubtedly good.

What you think is what you get.

Because here's the deal.

There is no absolute good or bad. There is nothing in the universe that says THIS is good and THAT is bad. *Humans* decide what is good or bad in the framework of their beliefs. What is seen as bad for one person might be perfectly acceptable for somebody else.

Remember…YOU GET TO DECIDE.

Imagine what your life would look like if you chose to believe that everything is good. Wouldn't you agree that when you are feeling thankful, you can't feel unthankful at the same time? It's humanly impossible

When you choose to practice gratitude toward everything in your life, you automatically shift a situation so that it becomes something to be appreciated – not because someone else has labeled it as such, **but because you have said that it is so.** You then bring forth all the goodness that is meant to be, in any situation, at any time, every single day of your life.

From this place, you live out what is stated in the quote – the acceptance, the order, the clarity, the gifts, and the perfect timing. You do this simply because you have chosen to do so.

Here's a perfect example.

I have two clients, both with a diagnosis of Polycystic Ovary Syndrome (PCOS), a health problem that can affect a woman's menstrual cycle and her ability to have children.

My first client, Elizabeth, was incredibly distraught after receiving the diagnosis from her doctor. She called me to complain and said, "This is the worse news! I really don't think this doctor knows what she's talking about! All I want to do is lose weight so that I go on this stupid trip, and now I have the added pressure of losing weight so that I can have a baby. There is just no way I can do this."

Elizabeth decided that having PCOS was bad. Her reality was that this new, more pressing reason to lose weight was going to keep her from getting to her desired results. This was too much for her to handle. Despite my efforts to coach her otherwise, Elizabeth called me the next week to say that she'd decided to stop seeing me.

When another client, Bethany, learned about her PCOS, she at first felt deeply saddened. She had tried several times to get pregnant without success. The PCOS confirmed that she would continue having trouble conceiving unless she corrected her diet.

Rather than continuing to feel sad, Bethany decided to take my coaching and feel thankful, even grateful, for the diagnosis.

"Julie, this was a total wake-up call," she said to me as she sat in my office. "If I hadn't known about the PCOS, I would have blamed all sorts of factors for my infertility. Now I know that if I want a baby, I need to recommit to everything we've been working on here."

Bethany realized that if she continued to work with me, shifting her diet with small changes every day, she could address the insulin resistance and other factors that were contributing to her condition.

Both women made a choice.

Elizabeth's choice to see the situation as bad kept her stuck in the Fat Kid Mentality that says, "It's okay to blame your weight on negative circumstances." Bethany's choice to practice gratitude allowed her to continue to heal and move toward other healthy behaviors.

At this point you may be thinking, "Okay, but how do I move into a place of gratitude every day?"

It's really much easier that you think.

Let's start now.

SMALL CHANGE:

Whenever my clients have a tough time practicing gratitude, I bring them through my Practice Gratitude Exercise. This is an incredibly effective tool for getting you to think less about what you are lacking and more about what you are blessed with.

Ideally, you should do this while you are alone in a quiet place that allows you to concentrate and really get present to your life.

Just let your thoughts and feelings flow. Be open to your process, without judgment, and with the intent to shift from the negative to the positive. You will be astounded at how quickly this shift happens.

1. Count Your Blessings

One way to get closer to gratitude is to focus on what is working, rather than what is not. When we focus on all that we have, then we naturally step into a place of gratitude.

Right now, make a list of ten things you are grateful for. This can be something as major as your family to something as minor as someone sending you a nice e-mail.

_____

_____

_____

_____

_____

_____

_____

_____

_____

_____

This list of ten may change every day. In fact, every night at dinner my family goes around the table and says three things they are grateful for. My son Max always says he's grateful for his parents. The other two things may be something like a toy, a friend, or the dinner we're having. It's always different. It's such a wonderful way to bond, and it really gets us present to what we have in our life, at that very moment, that inspires us to give thanks.

You can also keep the same list of ten and just refer to it every day as a reminder of your life's goodness.

THIS is practicing gratitude.

2. Say Thank You

Imagine what it would feel like to REALLY pay attention when you say the words "thank you" – even if to just thank the store clerk who is bagging your groceries.

When you thank someone, you are stating your appreciation for what that person has done for you. When you say these words with meaning, rather than doing it out of habit, you will be amazed at how that small gesture shifts feelings of lack into feelings of abundance.

Try this out with these simple steps the next time you are thanking someone:

    a. Smile or at least pay attention to your facial expression.
    b. Look the other person in the eyes as you say the words instead of fumbling in your purse for your cell phone or putting your credit card back in your wallet.
    c. Say the words more slowly, thus adding more intention.

Take note of how this made you feel. It can be like a shot of adrenalin. Now, this rush could be because you are creating a connection with someone, and that might make you nervous. Yet it's this connection to others that gets you more connected to yourself. In doing so, you move away from the chaos in your mind and find solace in the simple act of reaching out to others. You honor yourself by honoring others.

THIS is practicing gratitude.

3. Reassign the Bad to the Good

This is my favorite exercise. It is also one that takes the most courage and a willingness to let go of your beliefs and create a new paradigm that embraces gratitude.

I first want you to write down ten things that you see as bad in your life. For example, it could be a failed marriage, your weight, your parenting skills, or even the traffic on the way to work.

_____

_____

_____

_____

_____

_____

_____

_____

_____

_____

Now I want you to turn it around and list why these ten things are actually good and serving you in a way for which you are thankful.

For Example:

"The traffic on the way to work is good because it reminds me to slow down, and it gives me time in the morning to be alone. Thank you."

Or

"These extra fifteen pounds are good because they serve as the catalyst to keep seeking improved health and to live my best life. Thank you."

_____

_____

_____

_____

_____

_____

_____

_____

_____

_____

_____

_____

Once you have completed these exercises, keep referring to them daily. As said above, you may have new items to add to your list every day. If you'd like to see profound changes taking place in your life, then make this a daily habit. You will soon realize that YOU are in control of what your life looks like...and you choose to be thankful for it all.

THIS is practicing gratitude.

BIG IMPACT:

Remember Elizabeth?

She was the one who stormed out of my office saying that she couldn't handle the pressure of the PCOS diagnosis and how that was going to hold her back from losing weight and getting pregnant.

Well, Elizabeth called me a year after she left my practice and said she'd like to come in for a visit. Of course I agreed.

When we started talking, Elizabeth explained that over the past year she'd gained another twelve pounds and was having severe pain in her joints that kept her from exercising. This, along with not being able to conceive, had made her anxious and depressed, for which she was being medicated.

She admitted that before she left my office the year prior, she had been making progress with the work we were doing together. When she reflected on this, and how her life had taken a turn for the worse since then, she decided to take a closer look at her role in getting healthy.

I smiled at Elizabeth and said, "Welcome back. You have taken a big leap of faith here, and that is to be commended. Now, are you ready to change your beliefs about everything that's happened in the last year?"

"I'm not sure what you mean," she said. "What beliefs?"

"Elizabeth, you are still stuck in the belief that everything in your life is bad. And from this place you are going to get upset every time I challenge you with something that feels uncomfortable or incongruent with what you believe will get you the results you desire."

She nodded.

"So we're going to start with an exercise that I know will move you out of the Fat Kid Mentality that keeps you in a pattern of blaming. Are you willing to do that?"

She said yes, so we dove in.

We sat together for the rest of her session and came up with all the things she was grateful for. I could tell she enjoyed this exercise, shyly smiling as she shared the joy she gets from her pets, her husband, her home, and even her favorite tabloid magazine that she looks for in the mail every week. For thirty minutes Elizabeth was completely freed from the pain and trials of the past year, instead basking in the warm glow of all the wonderful things life had bestowed on her.

With this vital energy, Elizabeth left my office with the assignment to complete the Practice Gratitude Exercise.

I saw Elizabeth the following week, and she shared her experience of turning the bad into good and what had transpired for her.

First, she said that the exercise had been easier than she'd expected. She was convinced she would list everything and get into a place of anger, sadness, guilt, and more blame.

Instead, knowing that she was writing the bad things down to **turn them around,** she felt inspired and excited about what she was going to come up with.

She first focused on the diagnosis of the PCOS, and wrote:

"The PCOS is good because it has taught me a huge life lesson on humility and the power our thoughts have over our health."

Wow. If that was all she'd written, that would have been sufficient. Her gratitude statement reflected a total transformation in Elizabeth's understanding of herself, as well as the relationship she had with her body.

Elizabeth was very present to this shift as well. She explained that this realization moved her out of the dieting mentality and into seeking total health and wellness despite her weight. She also launched a vigilant effort to control her thoughts, with the intent to turn bad into good every day.

We continued reviewing her list, and by the end our session Elizabeth was committed to making small changes every day in her thinking, her diet, and her exercise – measures that greatly increased her chances for getting pregnant the following year.

You see, you create your own story.

You can wake up every morning and write the plot for how your day is going to be. Start by practicing gratitude. When you do this, your story will always be filled with optimism, faith, and joy. Then, if the day turns out differently than you imagined, you have the ability to rewrite the ending – one that comes from a place of gratitude and thankfulness for the blessings that showed up in your life that day.

Wake up the next day and do it again. The next day, do it again.

Soon you will always be practicing gratitude. Imagine what that would create the next time you get on the scale or sit down for a meal or have a day where things didn't go the way you planned.

When you see all the events in your life as good, then you will feel more motivated to write a new story the next day. This way of thinking and acting is much more empowering than focusing on the negative, which will stop you in your tracks and keep you stuck in the Fat Kid Mentality forever...GUARANTEED!

So take a stand for yourself and for your life and practice gratitude. You will be so thankful that you did.

Daily Lesson #14:

ERADICATE THE FAT KID
MENTALITY IN CHILDREN

W hat is a fat kid?

The clinical definition is any child who has a Body Mass Index (BMI) in the 95th percentile of the pediatric growth charts.

My definition of a fat kid is every person who is programmed with the Fat Kid Mentality and suffers from limiting beliefs around food, exercise, and a negative self-view.

Take my client, Denise.

She has two children with varying needs around nutrition. Her younger son, Jason, is eight years old and obese. His biggest problem is portions. Her ten-year-old, Brian, is a "bean pole who can eat anything he wants." Since Brian's the skinny one, he gets away with drinking soda and eating fast food and always goes back for seconds.

When Denise walked into my office, she looked like she could break down at any moment. When I asked how I could best help her family, she said she'd start by telling me her own story around food.

"As a child I was skinny; my sister was the fat one," she began. "My parents would tell me to hide food from my sister so that she wouldn't eat it."

I empathized with her and thought how pissed off I would be if someone told me what to eat!

"Today, I know this affects how I treat food with my children," she admitted. "Jason is overweight, but he's so hungry all the time I don't want to deprive him of the food that he loves. I also don't want to make my older, skinnier son angry by limiting the food in our house so that the younger one won't eat it."

She went on to say that she doesn't impose any rules around food – that she gives her kids options and trusts they'll make good decisions.

Clearly this wasn't working. Unless a child is educated about his food choices, and how those choices impact the things that are important to him – e.g., grades, sports, social popularity – he will gravitate toward the food that gives him immediate gratification.

So by expecting a child to make healthy choices, without giving him compelling reasons for doing so, Denise was setting herself up for a losing battle. She disguised her discomfort around rules by giving her kids more rights, and in the process she disempowered everyone.

Denise is not alone.

And she is not a bad mom.

She is just stuck in the Fat Kid Mentality that says, "Setting rules around food means deprivation."

In living out her patterns from childhood, Denise felt guilty every time she regulated her sons' portions and intake of sugar. Her motherly instincts told her to intervene. But her Fat Kid Mentality from childhood said, "If you do that you're depriving your kids, and that is unkind."

No mother wants to be unkind to her child. I get that. So I knew I needed to educate Denise about what was really going on.

Here's what happened next.

After a long pause I said, "Denise, when you give in to your kids' eating habits, you are depriving them of something much more precious than a hamburger or a bowl of ice cream.

"What you're really doing is depriving them of their health, their energy, their vitality, and their potential to live an awesome life.

"Tell me, what is Jason's life worth to you? Is it worth a little discomfort at the dinner table when you say, 'We're not having dessert tonight'? Is it worth some resistance from Brian when you limit snacks and sweets? Is it worth taking a deeper look at your own beliefs around food so that you don't pass on this defeating cycle?"

Denise looked at me and with a deep knowing said, "Yes, it's all worth it to me. I know I'm the one keeping everybody stuck."

I gave Denise a huge hug. What a brave act to admit her shortcomings and agree to relinquish the past to create a better future for her kids. I was so proud of her.

She admitted, however, that she was tired of trying to come up with solutions on her own. She needed help getting everyone on board with her goals for better health and had come to me to design a plan on which everyone could agree.

This was perfect! We signed her up for my Family Wellness Program and set an appointment for our first home-visit the following week.

Before Denise left, I set the foundation for the work we were going to do together. I explained the Fat Kid Mentality, and that not only she but both her boys were stuck in this limiting mindset.

As I was talking, she started to laugh and said, "Oh my gosh, you're right! We all have these crazy beliefs around food, and it's so ridiculous!"

I was happy for the levity and went on to explain that even though Jason has been described as the "fat" one with the BMI in the 95th percentile, Brian was also at risk.

You see, the BMI is misleading because it is just a height to weight ratio. It is not a direct measurement of visceral body fat – the dangerous kind that leads to disease.

For example, you have two boys standing next to each other, both in the 95th percentile. You can clearly see that one boy is lean and muscular and that the other boy has a fat belly that hangs over his jeans. Extra muscle adds to body weight, so the lean boy will register as overweight according to the charts but may just be a big kid with lots of muscle. The other boy will not only register overweight on the charts but will actually be a fat kid.

Jason clearly has extra body fat, coupled with eating junk food, not exercising, and engaging in negative self-talk. Unless we change his patterns, then he'll remain the fat kid destined to be a fat adult!

At the same time, Brian believes he is impervious to the sugar- and fat-laden foods that fill his diet. With these beliefs, he is still limiting himself with the Fat Kid Mentality that says, "I can eat anything I want."

Even though Brian is the skinny kid, his Fat Kid Mentality could still lead him down a dangerous road to ill-health.

Consider the views of pediatric cardiologist Reginald Washington, MD, who is the co-chair of the American Academy of Pediatrics Task force on Obesity.

Dr. Washington says that even if heavier kids are at greater risk for becoming heavy adults this does not mean a skinny kid will become a skinny adult. There are many predictors for obesity, but the easy availability of calorie-dense foods and increasingly sedentary lifestyles top his list of environmental influences contributing to what he calls a "global obesity epidemic."

University of Colorado professor of pediatrics, Dr. Nancy Krebs, MD, says the biggest predictor of whether a chubby baby will become an overweight child, teen, or adult is his parents' weight.

"As a physician, if I see an infant or toddler becoming overweight, I judge how worried I need to be by looking at the parent," she says.

I go even deeper.

Even if the parents are thin, like Denise, that doesn't mean they are raising healthy kids. If they are stuck in the Fat Kid Mentality, then they will negatively impact their children's eating habits by their own limiting thoughts.

So this Daily Lesson is for parents who want to end the cycle.

It's about saving the fat kid who is already struggling with weight and preparing for a lifetime of disappointment and ill health.

It is also for the *other* kid, whose unhealthy habits are creating a skewed physiology that could lead to obesity or other health conditions in adulthood.

In reality, this Daily Lesson is about saving every child from the Fat Kid Mentality before it sets unhealthy behaviors into motion. If you can teach your children – as a parent, a teacher, a caregiver – by using the lesson you learn today, you will be saving them from years of unhealthy behaviors.

The change starts with you – the adult.

Just like on an airplane when they instruct you to put on your oxygen mask before assisting your child, you need to help yourself first. You need to be healed, empowered, and free from the Fat Kid Mentality before you can save your child's life. Your kids are telling you how they feel about themselves by buying into unhealthy behaviors and ways of thinking. If *you* are buying into the Fat Kid Mentality, then you can bet they are buying in too!

You would walk through fire for your child. Let this Daily Lesson be your guide to a different future. In changing your own habits, you can now teach your children how to change theirs.

SMALL CHANGE:

Sit down with your children and have a family meeting. Be careful not to make it a serious meeting, which everyone will dread.

Rather, set it up in a positive light, letting everyone know you're making some changes, as a family, to promote healthier habits. Tell your kids you love them – with a smile. Laugh a little at your current situation, and include yourself as someone who, up until now, has not made the best choices.

It's also important to start with a small and tangible change, so as not to overwhelm everyone. Remember, if I had decided to run six miles my first day out, I would never have started. But I ran eight blocks, and it changed my life.

So don't plan to change everything all at once. You're a dead duck if you say:

"Okay, tomorrow we're doing things totally different around here! We're going to start eating breakfast, I'm cutting out all sugar, and no more treats for doing your homework. Oh yeah, and you need to start exercising."

If you can follow my philosophy of **Small Change, Big Impact**™, you'll find that the small changes will bring forth more changes, and then more changes, and so on.

So pick a change that is meaningful to you. If you feel that eating breakfast will have the biggest impact, then start there. If you feel your children need to focus on smaller portions, then start there. Or maybe you just want everyone to help with the meal planning.

Whatever you decide, THIS is what's perfect for you. Now, here's how to get your children on board with your vision.

An enrolling conversation could look like this (good for ages four to sixteen):

"Okay, guys, you know how I love to eat ice cream? Well, I read this book and I was asked to take a two-week sugar holiday. I did it and I feel awesome! It's important to me that you feel this good too. So on Sunday we're going to sit down and talk about what we can do to eat healthier. Don't

worry, I'm not taking away your favorite foods. I just want to share ideas on how we can cut back on sugar and reserve it for special treats rather than have it every night for dessert."

What you've done here is let everyone know that you committed to making a change, cut out the sugar, and now you feel great and want to share your experience. You are also not giving into the Fat Kid Mentality that says, "Sugar is bad." You are really saying that you've learned sugar is just something to be regulated, which will make them feel better. Most importantly, you are owning your role as parent and taking a stand for your kids so that they can live a healthy life.

Here's another conversation (good for ages seven to ten):

"So, Cameron, I've noticed you're watching lots of TV lately and not really paying attention to exercise. Believe me, I've had to make some changes around this too. But I found that I really love to swim. I used to hate exercise because I couldn't find anything that I enjoyed. What do you say we sit down tomorrow night and come up with ways to get you moving a little more – you know, find some activities that you'll enjoy. Maybe we can find some things we can do together."

In this conversation, you're not placing judgment on Cameron by saying, "You're not exercising enough." That kind of statement sets up the Fat Kid Mentality, essentially saying, "You're bad because you're watching TV and not exercising like everyone else." By giving Cameron options, you're also letting him know that exercise can be whatever he wants it to be – that he can identify what he likes and set his own pace and timeline. Lastly, by suggesting activities to do together, you show Cameron that his health is so important that you will devote part of your day to exercise with him.

And here's one more (good for ages six to sixteen):

"Hey, gang, would you agree that our mornings are a little crazy? It really bums me out that we're not getting our days off to a good start with breakfast. So on Thursday night we're going to sit down as a family and come up with a list of quick, easy breakfasts that we can all enjoy. It's up to me, as your parent, to make sure you're eating breakfast every day. But it's up to all of us to come up with ideas that we can agree upon so that eating breakfast can be easy."

By admitting that the house is a zoo in the morning, you let your kids know that this does not need to be the norm. Many times the Fat Kid Mentality is set up around chaos and the idea that this is just how life is. You can create a different reality for your kids. In addition, by getting everyone to help out with meal ideas, you teach personal responsibility so your kids don't blame their eating habits on their circumstances. You have also let them know that you're still in charge. You will still enforce breakfast but are giving them options with a family-designed list.

Once you get the family on a plan, commit to that plan for thirty days. Every day for the next month you need to show that this small, intentional change, performed with consistency, can create big impact results. Believe me, when your kids start to feel better, sleep better, behave better (with fewer consequences), and even lose weight (if needed), they will stay committed to that small change.

Once you have mastered that small change, schedule another family meeting to discuss the next small change. Sometimes it may take you more than thirty days to have the first small change fully integrated into your family culture. That's okay. As long as you commit to thirty days, your kids see that this is for real. It really takes only twenty-eight days to form a habit but, honestly, kids "get it" much faster than adults!

If you took on one small change every month, imagine what your family's health would look like at the end of one year.

Keep reading to see what that could create.

BIG IMPACT:

So here's what I did with Denise and her boys.

At the end of our first family meeting, I had each of them choose a small change that they could commit to until our next meeting, which was the following week.

Jason decided he would pay attention to portions. We used one of the handouts from my *Family Wellness Guidebook,* which shows portion sizes in relation to the size of your hand. Jason agreed to make his cereal, rice, and pasta portions equal to what he could hold in his cupped hand.

That was it. That's all he committed to.

Yes, he really needed to eat breakfast every day. Yes, he needed to stop using food as a reward. He also needed to eat more whole foods and start exercising more frequently. But that would have been too much for Jason to commit to all at once. So we chose one small change and started there.

Brian decided to stop drinking soda, and Denise chose to cut back her lattes to three days a week, rather than having one every day.

What a joy to see them the following week! They had stuck to their plan and all of them felt motivated to keep going. The next week was the same, and at the end of thirty days they had all stayed committed. By this time, they were ready for the next small change.

What was so cool was that by committing to the first small change, they started to break through some of their limiting beliefs around food and were making additional small changes without even trying.

By eating smaller portions, Jason naturally took in less sugar and found that he had more energy. He was having more fun at soccer practice and asked his mom if he could also join the lacrosse team.

Brian noticed he was sleeping better without all the soda and woke up earlier, which gave him more time in the morning to eat a healthy breakfast rather than grab a sugary doughnut. It helped that Denise wasn't keeping those foods in the house anymore but allowed them as special treats, three times a week, just like her morning lattes. When she realized she could moderate the sweets without feeling deprived, she knew her kids could too.

At the end of six months Jason had lost fifteen pounds. I never once put him on a scale. The only way I knew he had lost weight was from the doctor's reports. If I had focused on his weight, then I would have been supporting the Fat Kid Mentality that says, "Weight loss is the only measurement of success." But this was not what we were trying to accomplish with Jason. My teachings were designed with much more purpose than Jason losing weight. The work I did with Denise and her family was about transforming the Fat Kid Mentality that had plagued Denise for years and was threatening to send her kids down the same path.

I continued to work with Denise in my adult coaching program. Her patterns were a little more set, but she made breakthroughs every week, and her kids were the direct recipients.

Brian stayed off the soda and stopped telling everyone he could eat whatever he wanted. He still took more liberties than his brother now and again, but his thinking had changed. He no longer believed that being healthy was just about being thin. He now knew his food and exercise choices affected everything in his life.

This is what can happen with your family. Take this Daily Lesson and pay it forward to the ones you love most – your children. They will thank you.

Final Chapter

PLAY ON THE COURT OF LIFE

You have just learned the fourteen powerful lessons to transform your Fat Kid Mentality.

Now it's time to go out and play on the court of life.

This is your moment. You are in a powerful space of optimism and knowledge. You have learned new ways of being, thinking, speaking, and believing. Now you can create a life of health, fitness, and vitality.

But notice that I used the phrase "learned new ways." It is yet to be seen that you will actually "live new ways."

You have a choice to make now – a road you must follow.

You see, this final chapter is the most important lesson in the book. It is the deciding moment that poses the question:

"Are you going to take the path that leads you toward doubt, fear, and old messages?

Or are you going to move into a new realm – the realm that is meant for you, the one that is calling you, the realm that has been there for you since birth?"

The life you envision is already yours. This book is no accident. Reading this book is something you created so you could move beyond life as you know it. Deep down, you know the life you want awaits you. Just reach out...you can touch it!

Consider that whoever recommended this book to you is your savior. This person was put in your life to make sure you read this book so you could set yourself free from the **Fat Kid Mentality** that has kept you stuck in ill-health for so long.

Yet even with the support of this book, the choice is still yours. It is your responsibility to take what you've learned and apply it to your daily life, to your world, to your very Being.

You need to cross the line of distinction – where on one side of the line you keep doing what you're doing now and on the other side you walk into the world of what's possible. My advice is that it's imperative to move away from the trappings of your old ways and design your life around these fourteen powerful lessons.

You can do this by following my Three D's to Success: **Decide, Declare, Do.**

Here's how you do it:

1) **Decide:** You need to decide today if you are ready to take on the fourteen powerful lessons and make them your own. This doesn't mean you need to do all of them at once – remember, Small Change, Big Impact™. All I'm asking is that you decide YES or decide NO. If YES, then go on to #2.

If NO, then here is my recommendation. You are just not ready for this information yet. That is okay. I really do believe in divine timing, and I know with conviction that this book has been placed in your life for a reason. So, please just set this book aside for sixty days. Don't touch it, don't refer to it, don't recommend it to anyone. Then in sixty days I want you to re-read it, and see if your decision is different.

2) **Declare:** Words are so powerful! Your decision of YES will have only as much power as you assign it. If you state your YES with clarity, strength, and conviction, then your life WILL SHOW UP with clarity, strength, and conviction. If you state your YES with apprehension and caution, then your action steps will reflect this apprehension and caution. How has this been working for you so far? State your intentions loud and clear with ALL THAT YOU'VE GOT! Write them down in a journal. Call a friend right now and declare your YES! Paste it on a vision board with pictures and words that illustrate what you want your life to look like in one year.

Clearly declare, "YES, I have changed my life, and I've taken on the powerful lessons in this book to eradicate the Fat Kid Mentality and manifest total health and wellness with ease."

3) **Do:** Now you must perform the Small Change action steps that I've placed before you. Did all of them resonate with you? Maybe not. But I know at least nine of the fourteen lessons spoke to you in a way that created a shift in your thinking. The shift will not last, however, unless you put the thoughts into action. *The thoughts are just the portal to change.* It would be like giving you food and telling you not to chew, swallow, or digest. **Ideas do not incur growth unless they are assimilated and assigned meaning to produce action.**

So here's what you must do. Go back to Daily Lesson #1 and, if you haven't already, incorporate breakfast into your life TODAY. Follow the Small Change actions steps for thirty days until eating breakfast becomes habit. If you've already solidified this habit during the course of reading this book, then move on to Daily Lesson #2. Keep moving through the lessons until they become so much a part of who you are that you can't imagine giving them up. They become sacred, something to be protected and cherished.

If you get stuck on one lesson, move on to the next one and give yourself a time frame to return and try it again. Contemplation is just a natural step before taking action. It you stay in contemplation too long, that's not beneficial to your life. But if you contemplate with the intent to create action, then you are preparing yourself for success. Just remember, DO stands for **Desired Outcome.** Go get what you want!

Keep in mind, life will get in the way of what you're setting out to accomplish. And not to be too cliché but...that's life. Work, kids, vacations, parties, crummy weather, too much laundry...these events are still going to happen. But rather than seeing them as roadblocks, embrace them as the natural unfolding of your life. That way you can liberate yourself from the idea that you need to be perfect. Because life is not perfect.

In fact, get a little messy! Life is messy (thank goodness), which allows for growth and the chance to have a little fun with this. I truly admire how kids can just jump in puddles of rain and not worry about getting muddy. They can eat an ice cream cone and have zero regard for the chocolate running down their face. They can paint a picture and see a masterpiece whereas others might see a blob.

Getting messy and not being perfect translate to having fun and creating your best life! You will mess up! Awesome.

When you mess up, that means you're playing the game, living on the court of life.

When you mess up you are taking a stand for yourself and deciding that today you are a living, breathing example of renewed hope and vigor.

When you mess up you are eradicating the Fat Kid Mentality that says, "I can't do this" and replacing it with a mentality that says, "I can do this – and I am!"

You know why?

Because when you mess up, YOU ARE DOING IT.

Now get out there and make it happen! And know that I love you, I am rooting for you, and I am calling in your greatness right now. I can't wait to hear how it shows up.

Appendix A

DIET DIARY AND EXERCISE LOG

Please complete your Diet Diary / Exercise Log every day.

1. Make note of the time you wake up.

_____

_____

2. List and describe in detail all foods and drinks and include the amount of each. Make note as to whether the food was fresh, frozen, canned, raw, cooked, baked, fried, etc. Note the time of each meal or snack. Be sure to list everything you eat or drink, including any condiments used (e.g., mayonnaise, mustard, relish, etc.).

_____

_____

_____

_____

_____

_____

3. Keep track of how much water you drink and list the amount in ounces. Also note the type and amount of any other drinks you consume.

_____

_____

_____

_____

4. Write down any activity or exercise you engaged in and how long you did it.

_____

_____

5. Note any periods of relaxation and what kind of relaxation it was.

_____

_____

6. Note the time you fall asleep.

_____

Day: Date: Day: Date:

Wake up time:

Morning
Meal:

Time:

Snack:

Time:

Mid-Day
Meal:

Time:

Snack:

Time:

Evening
Meal:

Time:

Snack:

Time:

Water Consumed:
(in ounces)

Other DrinksConsumed:
(in ounces)
(those not listed with meals or
snacks above)

Activity/Exercise:

How long:

Activity/Exercise:

How long:

Relaxation
type:

How long:

Fall Asleep time:

Appendix B
PROTEIN SOURCES

Dairy & Dairy Alternatives	Serving	G Protein
Organic cottage cheese	1/2 cup	16
Organic kefir	1 cup	14
Organic plain yogurt	8 oz	12
Organic milk (2%, 1%, skim)	1 cup	9
Goat feta cheese	2 oz	8
Organic string cheese	2 oz	14
Soy milk	1 cup	6
Almond milk	1 cup	3

Fish	Serving	G Protein
Fresh tuna	4 oz	32
Halibut	4 oz	30
Flatfish, flounder or sole	4 oz	27
Rainbow trout	4 oz	27
Cod	4 oz	26
Orange roughy	4 oz	26
Salmon	4 oz	25
Tilapia	4 oz	23
Catfish	4 oz	18
Light tuna, canned in water	3 oz	22
Salmon, canned	3 oz	18

Peas & Beans	Serving	G Protein
Edamame (Soy beans)	1/2 cup	11
Navy beans	1/2 cup	10
White beans	1/2 cup	9.5
Lentils	1/2 cup	9
Black beans	1/2 cup	9
Kidney beans	1/2 cup	7
Lima beans	1/2 cup	6
Chick peas/Garbanzo beans	1/2 cup	6
Pinto beans	1/2 cup	6
Black-eyed peas	1/2 cup	6
Green peas	1/2 cup	4
Hummus	3 Tbsp	3

Eggs	Serving	G Protein
Eggs	1 large	6
Egg whites	1 large	4

Meats	Serving	G Protein
Poultry* (chicken, turkey)	3 oz	25
* I don't recommend much poultry, but want to give you measurements until you've chosen a mostly plant-based diet. Please avoid beef, lamb and pork.		

Nuts & Seeds	Serving	G Protein
Soy nuts	1 oz	11
Peanut butter	2 Tbsp	8
Peanuts	1 oz (30 large)	7
Pine nuts	1 oz	7
Almonds	1 oz (23 nuts)	6
Almond butter	2 Tbsp	6
Pistachios	1 oz (50 nuts)	6
Mixed nuts	1 oz	5
Walnuts	1 oz (14 halves)	4
Pecans	1 oz (20 halves)	3
Cashews	1 oz	4
Sunflower seeds	1 oz	4

Meat Substitutes	Serving	G Protein
Tempeh	4 oz	21
Tofu	4 oz	20
Vegetarian burger	1 patty (2.5 oz)	13

Vegetables & Grains	Serving	G Protein
Artichokes	1 cup cooked	5.9
Asparagus	1 cup cooked	5.3
Beet greens	1 cup cooked	3.7
Beets	1 cup cooked	2.7
Broccoli	1 cup cooked	4.5
Brussels sprouts	1 cup cooked	5.5

Vegetables & Grains	Serving	G Protein
Cauliflower	1 cup cooked	5.3
Sweet corn	1 cup cooked	4
Mushrooms	1 cup cooked	3
Quinoa	1 cup cooked	12
Brown rice	1 cup cooked	7
Whole grain bread	2 slices	7
Millet	1 cup cooked	11
Barley	1 cup cooked	19
Oats	1 cup cooked	13
Amaranth	1 cup cooked	14
Salba®	2 Tbsp ground	2.5

Appendix C
SNACK AND MEAL IDEAS

Snacks:

- 1 peach with a handful of cashews or walnuts
- 1 rice cake topped with hummus and tomato or 2 teaspoons of peanut butter
- 10 almonds with 2 cups of air-popped popcorn
- 8 ounces of Greek yogurt mixed with blueberries or 1 small banana
- 1 cup steamed edamame sprinkled with sea salt
- 1 hard-boiled egg mashed with shredded carrots and served on whole-grain crackers
- 2 sticks of string cheese with a 2 tangerines or 3 apricots
- ½ cup cottage cheese with one cup of berries or served on top of salad greens
- A whole-wheat English muffin topped with baby spinach, hummus and ¼ avocado
- Smoothie – Blend 1 scoop protein powder (Juice Plus® + Complete) with 1 cup frozen fruit and water or ¼ cup juice.
- 3 ounces deli turkey slices wrapped around roasted asparagus or grilled veggies
- 1 apple with 2 tablespoons peanut butter
- 1 cup slow-cooked oatmeal topped with ½ cup mango, sprinkled with almonds

Tasty Tortilla Toppings:

Add these toppings to your favorite whole wheat tortilla (or for those avoiding gluten, use a gluten-free tortilla or a romaine lettuce leaf) – roll and enjoy!

- 2 tablespoons ricotta cheese mixed with ½ cup sliced
  or mashed strawberries
- ¼ cup hummus w/slices of cucumber, green-leaf lettuce,
  tomato, and avocado
- 2 tablespoons almond or peanut butter with sliced banana
- 2 tablespoons cashew or hazlenut butter sprinkled with raisins
- 2 tablespoons mashed black or pinto beans with melted
  low-fat cheese and salsa
- ¾ cup tuna salad with sprouts, baby spinach, tomato
  and sweet pickle relish
- 2 ounces sliced turkey, avocado, and sauteed mushrooms
- 2 ounces feta cheese topped with shredded zucchini
  and warm marinara sauce
- ¼ cup guacamole with shredded carrot, cabbage,
  and salsa
- ½ cup egg salad – 2 hard-boiled eggs, 2 teaspoons mustard,
  dash salt
- ½ cup low-fat cottage cheese, tomato slices, sprinkled
  w/sunflower or pumpkin seeds
- ¼ c. brown rice with roasted red peppers and drizzled
  with basil pesto
- 2 ounces turkey slices, 3 cooked asparagus spears,
  sprinkle w/Italian dressing
- ¼ cup avocado bean dip – blend 1 15-ounce can northern
  beans (drained) with 1 ripe avocado, ¾ cup salsa, 2 tablespoon
  lemon juice and dash sea salt
- 3 ounces grilled halibut with pico de gallo
- 2 scrambled eggs, feta or shredded low-fat cheddar,
  cooked broccoli and salsa
- 3 ounces baked tofu with ½ cup brown rice and tamari sauce

Meals:

Breakfast:
- 1 cup of slow-cooked or steel-cut-cooked oatmeal, 1 tablespoon chopped or ground walnuts and ½ cup blueberries, with ½ cup low-fat plain yogurt or soy milk.
- 2-egg omelet made with 1 whole egg and 1 egg white, veggies of your choice, e.g., ½-1 cup broccoli, mushrooms, tomatoes, etc., 1 slice of whole wheat toast, 1 cup cubed melon
- Smoothie – 1 scoop protein powder (I recommend JuicePlus+® Complete), 2 teaspoons honey, ½ a frozen banana, ½ cup blueberries, ½ cup coconut or almond milk, ½ cup water, 1 tablespoon Salba®, and 1 handful spinach or kale for extra health benefits.

Lunch:
- Large bowl of salad greens, such as romaine or baby spinach, topped with 2 ounces pumpkin seeds or walnuts, ½ cup kidney beans (or black or pinto beans), ½ of a sliced red or orange pepper, 1 tablespoon olive oil with 2 tablespoons balsamic vinegar or red wine vinegar, 3 whole-grain crackers or ½ of a pita bread
- 3-ounce turkey burger or 2 veggie burgers topped with 2 slices of avocado, 1 slice tomato, and 1 lettuce leaf, on a whole wheat English muffin
- 1 cup of lentil or black bean soup, with a salad made of arugula, cherry tomatoes, 2 tablespoons crushed walnuts, ¼ of an avocado, freshly squeezed lemon and/or 1 tablespoon balsamic vinaigrette salad dressing.

Dinner:
- 4 ounces poached or baked salmon (wild salmon is preferred over farmed salmon) served with 1 cup steamed broccoli topped with lemon juice, 2/3 cup cooked quinoa or brown rice – you can also substitute grains for 1 baked sweet potato.
- 4 ounces organic rotisserie chicken served with ½ cup cooked brown rice or ½ baked potato and 1 cup steamed broccoli or kale

drizzled with 1 teaspoon olive oil or lemon juice and just a dash of salt and pepper.

• Tempeh fajitas – 4 ounces tempeh stir-fried with ½ red bell pepper, ½ green bell pepper, and ¼ cup onions, all sliced – sprinkle mixture with ½ teaspoon. cumin, ½ teaspoon chili powder, and ¼ teaspoon garlic salt, stir-fry or sauté until tempeh is warmed; serve with 2 corn or small whole wheat flour tortillas, 2 tablespoons chopped tomatoes, and ¼ avocado, sliced.

Appendix D
RECIPES

BROCCOLI WITH SUNDRIED TOMATOES

Serves about 6

1 pound broccoli
3 tablespoons balsamic vinegar
1 small garlic clove, minced
4 tablespoons extra virgin olive oil
2 sun-dried tomatoes, oil-packed, chopped
1 tablespoon pine nuts
Champagne wine vinegar
Salt and pepper to taste

Add water and a pinch of salt to a medium-size pot and bring to a boil. Meanwhile, rinse and chop broccoli, dividing stems from florets.

In a small bowl, whisk together balsamic vinegar, garlic, and olive oil.

When water is boiling, add broccoli stems for about 2 minutes and then add florets for an additional minute. Pour into colander and rinse under cold water to stop the cooking. Drain well.

Toss broccoli with sun-dried tomatoes, pine nuts, and vinaigrette. Add salt and pepper to taste and, if desired, an additional dash of champagne vinegar.

EASY CUCUMBER SALAD

Serves 6 to 8

3 large cucumbers, peeled, thinly sliced
1 cup vinegar – rice, champagne, or cider
3/4 cup water
3/4 cup honey
1 teaspoon salt
1/8 teaspoon black pepper
Dash ground cayenne pepper
Dash dried parsley flakes
Dash dried leaf basil

Combine all ingredients except cucumbers; heat until sugar melts. Pour warm mixture over cucumbers. Store covered in refrigerator.

HEALTHIER ARTICHOKE DIP

Yields 2 cups

1 14-ounce can artichoke hearts, drained
2 tablespoons olive oil
1/8 cup Parmesan cheese, grated
Juice of ½ lemon

Combine all ingredients in a blender or food processor and purée until well-blended. Serve this with a big platter of immune-boosting veggies that everyone will enjoy like carrot sticks, grape tomatoes, cucumbers, red peppers, broccoli, and lightly steamed green beans.

HEALTHY WALDORF SALAD

Serves 4

2 ½ cups chopped apple – Fuji and Gala are especially good
1 cup red grapes
1 cup diced celery
½ cup walnut pieces
½ cup raisins
1/3 cup Greek yogurt
1 tablespoon fresh lemon juice

Toss all ingredients in a large bowl, making sure all the ingredients are well coated. Served chilled – great for lunches too!

MAKE-AHEAD PUMPKIN CUSTARD

Serves 6

2 eggs, beaten
1 cup plain Greek yogurt
½ cup honey
2 cups canned pumpkin
1-2 tablespoons pumpkin pie spice

Preheat oven to 375 degrees. Purée all ingredients in processor or blender. Pour mixture into lightly greased glass baking dish. Bake for 45 minutes or until center is firm. Let sit for 15 minutes before serving.

I like this best when served chilled. Great for breakfast, snack, or dessert.

CHUNKY MINESTRONE
Serves 12

1 tablespoon olive oil
1 cup chopped onion
1 medium carrot, halved lengthwise and thinly sliced
2 cloves garlic, minced
1 14½-ounce can no-salt-added diced tomatoes, undrained
1 14-ounce can reduced-sodium vegetable broth
1 cup water
1/4 cup brown rice
1 teaspoon dried Italian seasoning, crushed
3 cups fresh baby spinach
1 15-ounce can no-salt-added navy beans, rinsed and drained
1 medium zucchini, quartered lengthwise and sliced (about 1½ cups)
1/4 teaspoon ground black pepper
1/8 teaspoon salt
Shredded Parmesan cheese (optional)

In a 4-quart Dutch oven, heat oil over medium-high heat. Add onion, carrot, and garlic; cook about 5 minutes or until onion is tender, stirring occasionally.

Stir in undrained tomatoes, broth, the water, uncooked rice, and Italian seasoning. Bring to boiling; reduce heat. Cover and simmer for 35 to 40 minutes or until rice is tender.

Stir in spinach, beans, zucchini, pepper, and salt. Return to boiling; reduce heat. Cover and simmer for 5 minutes more. If desired, sprinkle individual servings with Parmesan cheese.

CARROT PATTIES
Makes 16 patties

1½ cups grated carrot (3 carrots)
3/4 cup finely chopped celery (2 stalks)
½ cup grated onion (1 onion), squeezed of juice in cheesecloth
  or paper towel
1/4 cup Panko or whole wheat bread crumbs
2 large eggs, lightly beaten
½ cup fresh parsley
1 teaspoon coarse salt
1/4 teaspoon freshly ground pepper
½ cup plain lowfat Greek yogurt
Canola oil

Combine the carrot, celery, onion, bread crumbs, eggs, parsley, salt, and pepper in a medium bowl. Press about 1½ tablespoons mixture between hands to form sixteen 2-inch patties and place on a tray.

Place a large nonstick skillet over medium-low heat. Coat lightly with canola oil. Place patties in the skillet and cook until golden brown, 3 to 4 minutes per side. Transfer to a serving platter. Serve each with a dollop of yogurt.

About the Author

Julie Hammerstein has helped thousands of people take back their health by following a simple step-by-step plan that gets results. Through personal consultation and family coaching, she has created a winning formula that gets people to think differently about health so they will act differently to make healthier choices.

She penetrates the hearts of her clients when she reveals her own experience of growing up overweight. She shares her story of personal growth and the realization that it's not about what shows up on the scale but how we carry ourselves in the world.

Her motto is this: **Small Change, Big Impact**™. "By making small intentional changes every day, you can take powerful steps to change your life with big impact results." This is the message Julie shares in her coaching, keynotes and seminars and in the educational and entertaining DVD series *Max's Minutes: The A-Z's of Healthy Living,* which Julie produced with her son, Max. She is also the host of a weekly web-based TV show called *Real Nutrition Q & A* on the Real Mom TV and Mom TV networks.

Julie lives in Denver with her boyfriend Andrew and their two boys, Max and Kai. She is surrounded by loving friends and family.